Emerging Issues in Family and Individual Resilience

Series Editors
Amanda W. Harrist
Stephan M. Wilson

More information about this series at http://www.springer.com/series/13415

Julie M. Croff • Jason Beaman
Editors

Family Resilience and Recovery from Opioids and Other Addictions

Springer

Editors
Julie M. Croff
National Center for Wellness and Recovery
Oklahoma State University Center
for Health Sciences
Tulsa, OK, USA

Jason Beaman
Center for Health Sciences
Oklahoma State University
Tulsa, OK, USA

ISSN 2366-6072 ISSN 2366-6080 (electronic)
Emerging Issues in Family and Individual Resilience
ISBN 978-3-030-56957-0 ISBN 978-3-030-56958-7 (eBook)
https://doi.org/10.1007/978-3-030-56958-7

This Springer imprint is published by the registered company Springer Nature Switzerland AG
The registered company address is: Gewerbestrasse 11, 6330 Cham, Switzerland

Preface

The American opioid epidemic brought national attention to substance use disorders. Changes in new product availability and opioid marketing resulted in increased rates of opioid prescribing in the late 1990s and early 2000s. These prescribing practices alone drove the first wave of the American opioid epidemic, which lasted for over a decade.[1] Trends in opioid prescribing peaked nationally in 2012; however, strength of opioid prescriptions remains about three times higher than it was in 1999.[2] By 2018, one in three Americans knew someone with an opioid use disorder;[3] this expansion of the profile of substance use disorders resulted in a widespread awareness for the family and other inter-personal effects of substance use disorders.

The role of family and community systems in recovery from substance use disorders (SUD) is robust and multifaceted. In the subsequent chapters, the authors share qualitative and quantitative evidence supporting strategies to increase resilience and recovery in family systems, workplaces, and communities, and across the life course. Chapters 1 and 4 focus on different aspects of women with substance use disorders in pregnancy. In Chap. 1, Dr. Qato shares dynamic and robust stories of stigma and bias for pregnant women who seek treatment for their substance use disorders. Critical gaps in care illustrated in Chap. 1 have an adverse effect on functioning of offspring, as described by Dr. Ciciolla in Chap. 4. Dr. Ciciolla describes improvements in treatment for mother and baby under circumstances of prenatal opioid exposure. Taken together, care provision suggested in Chaps. 1 and 4 can improve the quality of life for mothers and their infants.

---

[1] Centers for Disease Control and Prevention (CDC). Vital signs: overdoses of prescription opioid pain relievers—United States, 1999–2008. MMWR Morbidity and Mortality Weekly Rep. 2011 Nov 4; 60(43):1487–1492.

[2] Centers for Disease Control and Prevention. Vital Signs: Changes in Opioid Prescribing in the United States, 2006–2015. MMWR 2017; 66(26):697–704.

[3] American Psychological Association. APA Public Opinion Poll – Annual Meeting 2018. March 23 – 25, 2018. Accessed June 23, 2020. https://www.psychiatry.org/newsroom/apa-public-opinion-poll-annual-meeting-2018

In Chap. 2, Jonathan Rosen does identifies how workplaces can protect employees from opioid use disorders. This chapter illustrates the importance of interpersonal and policy practices where people in the United States spend the majority of their time: at work. Workplaces are the major source of health insurance in the United States; therefore, as institutions, workplaces control access to substance use treatment. Robust plans to pay for the treatment of substance use disorder are an important part of recovery. Finally, this chapter highlights how substance use disorders, particularly in the context of prescription opioids as a result of a workplace injury, should be treated like any other on-the-job injury.

Chapter 3 expands upon our understanding and the need for prevention. First introduced by Rosen as ways of avoiding workplace injury, Dr. Rezapour and colleagues explore prevention of substance use disorders in adolescence and early adulthood. The approach of these authors is critical for delaying first use. Key to this approach is identification and treatment of underlying mental health problems, in order to avoid negative reinforcement through substance use.

Dr. Hays-Grudo and colleagues expand our understanding of the role of early life adversity in Chap. 5. This chapter explores the transmissibility of substance use disorders through epigenetics, behavior, and other exposures (including prenatal exposure). Notably, Hays-Grudo emphasizes the importance of prevention of early life adversity and the ability to heal and grow from those early experiences. Notably, recovery from early life adversity is emphasized as an important component of therapeutic treatments for substance use disorders.

Recovery capital is another important component of treatment outcomes. In Chap. 6, Dr. Cleveland and colleagues define and describe recovery and recovery capital, as well as the importance of aligning our measurement, theory, and practice to improve treatment outcomes. Recovery capital critically includes family systems as part of a context and environment that fosters recovery.

The unique gifts given from parents to children are passed through generations. Dr. Robbins shares insight into a multi-generational approach for the prevention of substance use disorders for American Indian, Alaskan Native, and other Indigenous populations in Chap. 7. This insight into healing our communities emphasizes how current actions may impact offspring seven generations in the future. This emphasis on connection to one's ancestors and descendants relates to the historical trauma experienced by American Indian, Alaskan Native, and other Indigenous populations in the United States, their loss of ancestral land, the forced migrations, the removal of children from American Indian, Alaskan Native, and other Indigenous families until 1978, and the use of alcohol and other drugs to escape feelings associated with these losses.

Finally, in Chap. 8, Dr. Brashaw and colleagues explore recovery in the context of caregivers and family members for those with substance use disorders. Dr. Bradshaw and colleagues' work emphasizes the importance of including family units in therapeutic approaches. The work presented demonstrates clearly the damage done through environmental exposure to individuals with substance use disorder. By improving treatment modalities and including therapeutic approaches for family members, systems can improve upon the treatment of pain and trauma in the family unit.

Taken together, these chapters illustrate the role of family systems in the development and treatment of substance use disorders. Family systems approaches can be used to prevent and treat early life adversity in order to reduce transition to substance use disorders, through identification and treatment of mental illness, and through worksite programming. Pregnant women and other family members should have access to high-quality treatment services and allowed to room-in in order to reduce the rates of neonatal abstinence syndrome and enhance neurodevelopment. Finally, recovery capital should be fostered through engaging family systems and culturally appropriate intergenerational approaches. Recovery from substance use disorders requires resilient, engaged family systems.

Tulsa, OK, USA

Julie M. Croff
Jason Beaman

Acknowledgments

We would like to thank Victoria Hui Holloman for her efforts in coordinating with the editors and authors. Her efforts are a major contribution to this completed book. We would also like to thank the Center for Family Resilience Research Associates and breakout box participants for their help in completing this volume: Dr. Catherine Curtis, Bonhak Koo, Dr. Kara Kerr, Dr. Amanda Morris, Dr. Alexander Mach, Dr. Colony Fugate, Dr. Michael Criss, Dr. Todd Spencer, Dr. Valerie Blue Bird Jernigan, Cassandra Camp, Dr. Valerie McGaha, Dr. Karina Shreffler, Christine Joachims, Scott Fry, Kris Stallard, Elizabeth, and Dr. Steven Ray Byers.

Contents

Contributors

Samantha Addante Department of Psychology, Oklahoma State University, Stillwater, OK, USA

Mira Armans Department of Psychology, Oklahoma State University, Stillwater, OK, USA

Shervin Assari University of Medicine and Science, Los Angeles, CA, USA

Spencer D. Bradshaw Human Development and Family Studies Department, Utah State University, Logan, UT, USA

Timothy R. Brick Department of Human Development and Family Studies, The Pennsylvania State University, University Park, PA, USA

Lucia Ciciolla Department of Psychology, Oklahoma State University, Stillwater, OK, USA

Julie M. Croff National Center for Wellness and Recovery, Oklahoma State University Center for Health Sciences, Tulsa, OK, USA

Hamed Ekhtiari Laureate Institute for Brain Research, Tulsa, OK, USA

Gina Erato Department of Psychology, Oklahoma State University, Stillwater, OK, USA

H. Harrington Cleveland Department of Human Development and Family Studies, The Pennsylvania State University, University Park, PA, USA

R. Steven Harrist Oklahoma State University, Stillwater, OK, USA

Jennifer Hays-Grudo Oklahoma State University Center for Health Sciences, Tulsa, OK, USA

Thomas G. Kimball Texas Tech University, Lubbock, TX, USA

Namik Kirlic Laureate Institute for Brain Research, Tulsa, OK, USA

Kyler S. Knapp Department of Human Development and Family Studies, The Pennsylvania State University, University Park, PA, USA

Amanda Sheffield Morris Oklahoma State University, Tulsa, OK, USA

Danya M. Qato School of Pharmacy and School of Medicine, University of Maryland, Baltimore, Baltimore, MD, USA

Ashley Quigley Department of Psychology, Oklahoma State University, Stillwater, OK, USA

Erin L. Ratliff Oklahoma State University, Tulsa, OK, USA

Tara Rezapour Institute for Cognitive Science Studies, Tehran, Iran

Rockey Robbins Jeannine Rainbolt College of Education, University of Oklahoma, Norman, OK, USA

Jonathan Rosen AJ Rosen & Associates LLC, Schenectady, NY, USA

Sterling T. Shumway Texas Tech University, Lubbock, TX, USA

Bryan Stare University of North Carolina, Charlotte, OK, USA

Jasmin Vassileva Department of Psychiatry, Institute for Drug and Alcohol Studies, Virginia Commonwealth University, Richmond, VA, USA

About the Editors

Dr. Julie M. Croff Executive director of clinical and population research at the National Center for Wellness and Recovery (NCWR) and a Professor in the Department of Rural Health at Oklahoma State University Center for Health Sciences. Text description of job should also be changed as indicated in the comment box. In her role as executive director, she oversees the strategic development and oversight of clinical research and population health research and programs for NCWR and is dedicated bringing hope to individuals and families affected by pain and substance use disorders. Previously, she served as the founding director of the MPH program at Oklahoma State University. Dr. Croff's research focuses on perinatal substance use and co-occurring exposures among diverse cohorts of women. She is currently the principal investigator of several NIH-funded projects. Among them, the planning phase of the Healthy Brain and Child Development (HBCD) study, a longitudinal research project which seeks to better understand the role of prenatal exposures on neurodevelopment; A COVID-19 study, which seeks to understand how social and economic consequences of COVID-19 response affect mothers with substance use disorders compared to those without substance use disorders; and the Tulsa FAB Study, which seeks to explore the interaction of substance use and dietary behavior in the periconceptional period. Dr. Croff has published widely in the area of alcohol and other drugs across multiple vulnerable populations. She received her Ph.D. in public health, with emphasis on health behavior, from the joint program at the University of California San Diego and San Diego State University. She received her master's degree in public health with emphasis on social and behavioral sciences from Boston University and her bachelor's degree in biology from San Diego State University.

Dr. Jason Beaman graduated medical school from Oklahoma State University Center for Health Sciences. He then completed simultaneous residencies in psychiatry and family medicine. After residency, Dr. Beaman completed a fellowship in forensic psychiatry at Case Western Reserve University in Cleveland, Ohio. He holds board certifications in family medicine, psychiatry, forensic psychiatry, and addiction medicine. After his fellowship, Dr. Beaman completed a master's degree in pharmacology with an emphasis in forensics at the University of Florida. He also obtained a master's degree in public health from Johns Hopkins University. Dr. Beaman currently serves as the chair of Psychiatry and Behavioral Sciences at Oklahoma State University Center for Health Sciences, as well as the executive director of Training and Education at the National Center for Wellness & Recovery at OSU Medicine.

About the Series Editors

Amanda W. Harrist received her Ph.D. in child and family studies from the University of Tennessee, Knoxville. She is currently a professor of human development and family science at Oklahoma State University, where she is also Associate Director for Education and Translation at the Center for Family Resilience and an Administrative Core Director for the Center for Integrative Research on Childhood Adversity (CIRCA). Her research is focused on understanding psychosocial risk and protective processes in children's social contexts, particularly the parent–child relationship and peer relations at school.

Stephan M. Wilson is currently the interim dean of the College of Education and Human Sciences and previously served as the dean of the College of Human Sciences. He is a Ph.D. in child and family studies from the University of Tennessee, Knoxville. He is an NCFR fellow, Fulbright fellow, regents professor at Oklahoma State University, legend recognition of the American Association of Family and Consumer Sciences, and has numerous teaching, research, and community engagement recognitions. His areas of expertise include cross cultural family science and adolescent social competence.

Chapter 1
Barriers to Care for Pregnant Women Seeking Substance Use Disorder Treatment

Danya M. Qato

The substance use crisis has exerted an unprecedented toll on communities and health systems across the United States. Pregnant women and newborns are particularly vulnerable to the adverse consequences of addiction and substance use, including of opioids. From 2000 to 2009, opioid use among pregnant women increased from 1.2 to 5.6 per 1000 hospital births, and the incidence of neonatal abstinence syndrome has increased 400% nationally in the past decade (National Institute on Drug Abuse 2019). While a vast armamentarium of resources has been leveraged to address this public health predicament, there remain critical gaps in access to care. We know little about the primary determinants of treatment access among substance-using pregnant women, especially at the city, state, and regional level. This may be due, in part, to the lack of emphasis on identifying and addressing the complexity of disparities—such as those due to stigma, racism, income and insurance status, and education—that inform trajectories of addiction and dispossess vulnerable pregnant women of necessary healthcare. Over 90% of substance-using adults delay or do not receive specialized treatment for their substance use disorder (US Department of Health and Human Services 2016), and slightly less than half of pregnant substance-using women receive recommended treatment—medication-assisted treatment (MAT) (Krans et al. 2019). Understanding who these women are and why they remain outside the healthcare system is critical to enable efforts at improving access to and equity in care and thus enhancing health outcomes for themselves and their children.

In this brief chapter, I present a literature review to explore the role stigma, racism, and other sociodemographic, structural, and political determinants play in challenging access to healthcare for vulnerable pregnant women who are substance users. In addition, I also share preliminary findings from qualitative interviews

D. M. Qato (✉)
School of Pharmacy and School of Medicine, University of Maryland, Baltimore, Baltimore, MD, USA

J. M. Croff, J. Beaman (eds.), *Family Resilience and Recovery from Opioids and Other Addictions*, Emerging Issues in Family and Individual Resilience,
https://doi.org/10.1007/978-3-030-56958-7_1

about barriers to care with healthcare providers and women who self-identify as being current or formerly pregnant substance users.

1 Literature Review

1.1 Problematizing Stigma

Research related to the impact of stigma on healthcare access and adherence to care is abundant. Broadly defined, stigma is a "powerful social process of devaluing people or groups based on a real or perceived difference" (USAID, Health Policy Project 2011). Stigma enables varieties of discrimination that ultimately deny the individual or group full social acceptance, reduce the individuals' opportunities (Goffman 1963), and fuel social inequalities (Parker and Aggleton 2003). Stigma is an often-cited barrier to healthcare access and adequate engagement among vulnerable groups, especially those engaged in behavior that is socially and legally constructed as "undesirable," for example, men who have sex with men and illicit substance users. For women who are pregnant and substance users, the impact of stigma on access to care can be overwhelming and definitive in informing whether or not they seek prenatal care and/or substance use disorder treatment or choose to engage with the healthcare system and healthcare providers at all. Part of the adverse impact of stigma derives from the fear women have of being mistreated by healthcare providers due to substance use. This fear may be founded based on their own lived experiences with the healthcare system and/or narratives of experiences of those in their social networks. In a paper aptly titled "The Giving Voice to Mothers study: inequity and mistreatment during pregnancy and childbirth in the United States," authors note that one in six women reported being mistreated during the course of their prenatal or labor care (Vedam et al. 2019). Forms of mistreatment included being shouted at or scolded by healthcare providers, being ignored, violations of privacy, withholding of treatment options, and sometimes even physical abuse. This mistreatment is pervasive in healthcare and, especially for Black women and other women of color, reinforce alienation from the healthcare system broadly.

Some theorists have pointed to the imperative to conceptualize stigma as a racialized concept that reproduces structural inequalities and mirrors the prevalent racism that is encoded in all health interactions in the United States (Howarth 2006). Parker and Aggleton suggest that health advocates, "move away from psychological models that see stigma as a thing which individuals impose on others and instead emphasize, the broader social, cultural, political and economic forces that structure stigma" (Stangl et al. 2019). These forces can include economic forces, like low-wage work, and interconnected ever-present forces like racism. It is helpful to consider this framing, especially when thinking through potential interventions that support access and promote equity and justice in healthcare systems that all too often reify the underlying racist political and social landscapes within which they are embedded and implicated.

1.2 Punitive Legal Frameworks

Legal environments play a significant role, though not fully defined, in whether or not pregnant women access care. Underlying the fear related to stigma, many state-level approaches to ostensibly mitigate fetal drug exposure and reduce substance use among pregnant women have been punitive in nature. There is no unified dataset that collects information on the number of pregnant substance users who have been incarcerated, lost custody of their child or children, or were otherwise criminalized as a result of substance use. One recent estimate by Paltrow and Flavin, considered an undercount, showed that illicit drug use was invoked in 84% of cases in which pregnancy was a "necessary factor leading to attempted and actual deprivations of a woman's physical liberty" (Paltrow and Flavin 2013). A highly criminalized environment often results in avoidance of healthcare among substance-using pregnant women rather than mitigation of substance use. Research has found that "women have reported that they delayed or avoided prenatal care altogether out of fear of punishment" (Stone 2015).

Other work has found that state and federal legislation, even while mandated broadly, is not enforced equally or consistently resulting in deeper and more entrenched racial inequities. The Child Abuse Prevention and Treatment Act (CAPTA) legislation, in particular, has been pointed to as further pushing women away from treatment. CAPTA is a broadly applied federal policy last reauthorized in December of 2010 that tied state receipt of federal grants to mandatory reporting of substance-exposed newborns and has played a significant role in barriers to care for substance-using pregnant women (Harfeld and Marlowe 2017). Further, previous limited research found MAT rates to be disproportionately lower in states with laws that permit child abuse charges for prenatal illicit drug use (Angelotta et al. 2016).

1.3 Racism

In a socio-ecological and legal environment where substance use is criminalized and stigmatized, and given entrenchment of racism, racial capitalism, and history of slavery in the United States, racism figures prominently as a barrier to healthcare access among pregnant, substance-using women. Specifically, given the systems of racial discrimination in which judicial and social services have been operationalized in the United States, it is no surprise that Black, Brown, and Indigenous women are most often targets of suspicion and punitive measures as it relates to substance use. According to the Centers for Disease Control and Prevention (CDC), maternal mortality rates are 4–5 times higher in these communities compared to white women (CDC 2019). Further, the CDC notes, "Even in states with the lowest pregnancy-related maternal mortality rates and among women with higher levels of education, significant differences persist. These findings suggest that the disparity observed in pregnancy-related death for Black and American Indian/Alaskan Native women is a complex national problem." This is cause for alarm and is directly related to experiences of individual, structural, and institutional racism in the healthcare process, irrespective of class. It is racism thus, not race, which is the primary predictor of maternal mortality related to constellation of factors that are both structurally and individually mediated. One paper (Saloner and Lê Cook 2013) noted that, even in treatment patterns, there are disparities in care:

> More than one-third of the approximately two million people entering publicly funded substance abuse treatment in the United States do not complete treatment. Additionally, racial and ethnic minorities with addiction disorders, who constitute approximately 40 percent of the admissions in publicly funded substance abuse treatment programs, may be particularly at risk for poor outcomes. Using national data, we found that blacks and Hispanics were 3.5–8.1 percentage points less likely than whites to complete treatment for alcohol and drugs, and Native Americans were 4.7 percentage points less likely to complete alcohol treatment.

Thus, research has shown that Black women and other women of color are less likely to both receive substance use disorder treatment and to be heard by healthcare providers. Moreover, among those who do enter treatment, these individuals are less likely to complete treatment as compared to their white counterparts. They are also more likely to die from pregnancy-related complications compared to their white counterparts, all else being equal. Advocacy organizations, specifically those led by black women such as Black Mamas Matter Alliance (2020), have focused their efforts on amplifying the role of racism in driving maternal mortality among Black women and of working toward person- and community-centered evidence-based healthcare solutions to address this crisis.

1.4 Access

The restricted number of providers able or willing to provide care, lack of treatment options available, and limited access to healthcare coverage have all negatively impacted women accessing care. A report by the Agency for Healthcare Research and Quality (AHRQ) noted that, especially in rural settings, engagement of primary care providers will be necessary in order to address the diverse number of patients who require MAT and the lack of providers providing therapy (AHRQ 2017). One paper found that in the general population of patients with opioid use disorder:

> During the decade from 2004 to 2013, use of treatment remained low for individuals with opioid use disorders and did not increase after accounting for changing population characteristics, underscoring substantial room for improvement. Individuals in treatment received care in more settings, with the greatest increases in inpatient treatment and at physician's

offices. Although physician's offices may provide access to buprenorphine, medication-assisted treatments are often unavailable in inpatient settings, which could hinder patient recovery (Saloner and Karthikeyan 2015).

A similar study investigated the predicament in states with high rates of opioid mortality (including Maryland) and found that "Many buprenorphine prescribers did not offer new appointments or rapid buprenorphine access to callers reporting active heroin use, particularly those with Medicaid coverage" (Beetham et al. 2019). The unrelenting challenge of providing holistic care for substance using pregnant women continues.

2 Findings from Respondents in Baltimore, Maryland

My interviews with respondents from the Baltimore, Maryland, area reaffirmed many of the barriers found in the literature. This ongoing work, which included both patient and provider perspectives, addresses gaps in our understanding of barriers to care for substance-using pregnant women and the distinct role legal and policy climates play in undergirding such barriers. Given an environment of increasingly limited resources, optimizing the translatability of public health research to effective policy and interventions by explicitly addressing patient concerns is of paramount importance. I sought to engage intimately with patient and provider communities in Baltimore City. Due to the higher prevalence of substance use and overdose compared to national rates, Maryland and neighboring states, like West Virginia, have been the epicenter of the national conversation regarding the substance use crisis. Because these geographic regions have among the highest rates of substance use in the United States, they are also most in need of critical context-specific, evidence-based interventions that can help stem the tide of the epidemic. In this pilot project and the preliminary analyses discussed in this chapter, I partnered with the Baltimore City Preventing Substance Exposed Pregnancies (PSEP) coalition, an arm of the B'more for Healthy Babies' citywide strategy, to improve birth to age 3 health outcomes.

The primary aim of this project was to explore the experiences, beliefs, and attitudes of healthcare providers and current and former substance-using pregnant women in Baltimore, Maryland, which affect this population's engagement with healthcare. I employed qualitative research methods via an iterative process of in-depth interviews to gather the depth and breadth of these women's experiences.

2.1 Methodology

Current and former substance-using (e.g., prescription opioids, heroin) pregnant women residing in the city of Baltimore and healthcare providers involved in their care were enrolled in this study. Study populations were derived through snowball sampling. I utilized a semi-structured interview schedule, developed collaboratively by the research team with patient feedback, to guide a conversation about individual patient and provider experiences related to fears, stigma, beliefs, attitudes, and barriers to care. Audio recordings were transcribed verbatim and participants were compensated for their time with a gift card. The transcripts were reviewed to identify major themes. My analysis followed the principles of grounded theory methodology (Glaser 1994), which is designed to develop a model for how groups of individuals interact, engage, and respond to a situation. I follow a constant comparative approach such that I compare newly coded data with previously coded data to ensure consistency as I develop the meaning of the codes. The study received approval from the Institutional Review Board of the University of Maryland, Baltimore.

This is an ongoing research project, and thus far in our interviews with five women who are Baltimore City residents and self-identify as being current or formerly pregnant substance users and two providers, the following themes have emerged with respect to articulating barriers to care.

2.2 *Autonomy and Harm Reduction*

One theme that emerged repeatedly among the providers and the women was the necessity to provide the space and support for women to feel respected with regard to autonomy over their bodies and thus adopt a harm reduction approach to care. One provider who is a practicing doula noted the importance of decentering the "addiction" when caring for pregnant women who are substance users. She said:

> Yes, her addiction may have a significant impact on her pregnancy, and her health and the health of her child, but at the same time, we do see the importance of that woman maintaining the autonomy over her body. And in that autonomy over her body, we have to give space for the fact that that means she may use [substances] and that we have to deal with that. You just cannot have one without the other…Because oftentimes, that could be the one key thing that gets her through this pregnancy, the old cliché, one day at a time…if that means counseling a women and saying, 'Okay, typically before you got pregnant you would use five times a day, can we get that down to three?' And be okay with it, because that is a vast improvement and it ripples into other areas of her life.

The doula notes that part of her care praxis is asserting this autonomy, "For me, what this means, is that the person has total autonomy over their body and over decisions they make about their body, including what they put in their body."

2.3 *Lack of Access*

Strategizing around entering a treatment facility due to the lack of space, one respondent noted how she admitted herself into a psychiatric unit, because she could not enter first into a residential center for pregnant women. She says, "When I found out I was pregnant, I went into a psych ward to stop using. And I didn't know I was pregnant and I told them I was suicidal, just to get treatment, because I couldn't get into a treatment center or a detox center at that specific moment, and I knew that a psych ward would help me detox." With only a few health clinics in the Baltimore area focused on caring for actively using pregnant women, including the Center for Addiction in Pregnancy (where this respondent eventually was treated), it is no surprise that this respondent would employ such an approach. Innovative ways of navigating into healthcare systems so that they may address the totality of your care are becoming more imperative as pregnant women are increasingly using different substances, not singularly opioids, and are finding it more difficult to engage in care as substance use treatment becomes increasingly siloed and myopically focused on opioids.

2.4 *Fear of State Involvement*

Fears of engagement with child social services agencies are a key driver for disengagement or lack of engagement with the healthcare system. One counselor recalls that:

> Some women who were pregnant didn't seek any kind of treatment or care until they had help with their addiction. So, for example, they avoided going to prenatal care because they didn't want to have to give urine because they didn't know what they tested the urine for, and they didn't want to have a paper trail- if they were still using. That could be used against them, if they did have their child taken at birth.

One counselor articulates this fear pointedly:

> I've worked with pregnant women and some, a lot of them, are scared by their doctors saying, 'Oh, your baby is going to be taken from you.' They don't have the actual education on what really happens and what is supposed to happen, and what the possibilities are. Just because somebody might make a report to CPS (Child Protective Services), doesn't mean your child is going to be taken.

The counselor goes on to say that one way to avoid this alarm is education of rights of the women in these encounters. They note, "So that's one thing I strongly believe in, is education for the population that's potentially affected by the mandatory reporting. To blindside someone who just gave birth to a baby in the hospital with a CPS worker showing up, I don't feel is right."

Lack of education around substance use treatment among care providers pronounces the stigma associated with care. Mandated reporting has also cultivated an environment of fear around these issues. The doula I interviewed noted the fear pregnant women have of retaliation by healthcare providers who are mandated to report and that the laws and the perceived laws around mandated reporting are often confusing. She says:

> Mandated reporting, to me, then becomes this hammer that practitioners then use to come down on women and it's not meant to be that way. I think mandated reporting, to me, is just

> a healthcare provider just reporting what they see and that's it. In reality, I think that it gets used as a hammer that just beats women down from first contact. She knows that even the minute she walks into a clinic, everyone that she comes into contact with, with a badge, is legally mandated to report her. So why would I go into a facility that every person that I come into contact with, is going to report me to somebody? How does that help? How is that harm reduction?

2.5 Co-occurring Mental Health Illness and Lack of Housing

Co-occurring and untreated or poorly treated mental health illness and lack of a consistent housing is a primary barrier to maintaining care and accessing care consistently. Given the context of increasing mental health diagnoses co-occurring with substance use, the imperative to incorporate psychiatric services into care is ever more urgent. One respondent, a 35-year-old Black mother who used heroin during pregnancy and sought treatment for addiction, says when asked about her mental health during pregnancy, "I was a mess. I was very, very depressed. I suffered from anxiety horribly. I suffer from PTSD from events that happened as a child, and mentally, I was not stable- at all." Further, the inability to consistenty access safe and affordable housing disrupts care and exacerbates adverse health outcomes associated with both mental illness and substance use.

2.6 Stigma

Both care providers and women expressed feelings of being "judged" for their decisions, even while in the care of health providers, and how that feeling impacted their well-being. When asked about the greatest barrier to care, one substance use counselor noted, "The first thing that comes to mind is stigma. The population I work with, specifically women with children who have substance use disorders, I know that's something they struggle with, and sometimes it becomes a barrier for treatment and for medical care for them. The fear of stigma and the fear of how people look at them."

A doula who was interviewed reaffirmed this situation:

> For women who are substance users, what we see is them not being treated simply as a pregnant woman. That goes back to how we focus and how we see any type of addiction. I think with a pregnant woman, the whole stigma attached to it becomes a burden to them. It makes them almost invisible and the only thing people are focused on is their addiction. So, I think our approach [to providing care] gets amplified that much more when we're dealing with a woman and her family, and that we don't necessarily focus on her addiction.

One respondent reflected on the microaggressions she encountered from healthcare providers at the hospital while she was in the throes of labor. She recounts how her feet were swollen, and "I would ask why my feet well up like that? And they would say, 'Probably because you used during pregnancy.' ...I said that can't be the reason. I said, 'Yeah, I used previously but I'm not using now, so why is it?' and they wouldn't have much to say...Some of it I would ignore, because I'm not going to entertain ignorance all the time." There is no doubt that such mistreatment permeates the healthcare system and impacts health outcomes, for the mother and the child.

2.7 *Self-Awareness*

Women had nuanced reflections about who they were via-a-vis the etiology of the addiction, the root causes of the addiction, as well as the potential resolution of it. Some women contextualized it as trauma. When discussing childhood events that adversely impacted her mental health, one respondent said:

> I definitely refer to it as trauma because it's impacted every aspect of my life. I didn't talk to anybody about it until I was in my early 20s. I held it in for all those years. I was like, very shameful of it, especially because my abuser had told me that if I was to tell anybody that my parents would want nothing to do with me, they'd be disgusted with me, and that I was to just keep quiet about it. And so that's what I did. And it just turned into a lot of anger as I got older.

One 35-year-old Black mother of four noted, "I'm mentally ill, due to trauma that I've been through as a child and through childhood and adulthood. Right now I'm getting to know myself, I really don't know who [I am] ...I'm an addict as well. I suffer from the disease of addiction and I'm determined to learn to live with my disease, being healthy and recovering until the day I die."

When asked what she meant by "addict", she goes on to say, "I'm an addict because I use things-not only drugs- I use things that make me feel normal, things that make me feel better about myself. It could be food, attention, that helps me cope with living. I say I'm an addict because I don't know how to deal with my feelings. I never had the help, professionally, to recover from the trauma I went through as a child."

She goes on to describe the types of trauma she experienced as an adult, including abandonment and verbal abuse. She describes the trajectory moving from alcohol to heroin to opioids and back and forth in perpetuity. Very clearly, she had been able to understand the multifaceted determinants of substance use disorder. The paternalistic structures of medical practice and provision often ignore and erase the reality that patients are often more well aware of their medical history than their own healthcare providers.

2.8 Lack of Awareness of Options Available

While it may seem counterintuitive, some respondents noted the preponderance of resources available at the city level and the parallel inability to thoughtfully navigate these resources as a barrier. One counselor noted the necessity of having a navigator on hand to help sort through what is available, "I think being connected to…a family preservation officer or if they have a good primary care doctor or if they have people who are willing to actually look at the needs that they have and try to help them address them. Otherwise, for them to just be like, 'Oh, I need housing and I don't even know where to start.' Or 'Who do I talk to? Where do I go?' If they're just dealing with that on their own and trying to navigate the system on their own, I think it's very easy for them to just give up. Just from feeling overwhelmed and frustrated."

2.9 Implications

Overall, many women pointed to a positive experience with their engagement with healthcare providers in specialty care. Women who received treatment at centers for addiction in pregnancy noted feelings of being respected and having autonomy over their healthcare situation. Providers noted the necessity to amplify autonomy of women over their bodies and to be gentle in providing care for substance using women, especially so when they are pregnant. One doula, when talking about her approach to caring for women, says:

> Women in general, our approach is gentle. We use the word gentle all the time, in how we approach women and their families. Gentle, open and supportive. Those are the three guiding principles in our training. Gentle, meaning that we see ourselves as an advocate, and not someone who's going to take over and give the women and the families we support these requirements they have to meet, in order for us to give them service. We take that away. There are no requirements, other than you say you want help. It's basically focused and generated on that specific client.

While few of the women interviewed specifically articulated feelings of being discriminated against, many felt that the specialized care that they received in fact allowed them to focus on caring for themselves and their babies (Breakout Box 1.1).

Breakout Box 1.1. Focus on Practice

As a registered nurse involved in opioid management among pregnant patients who also has the personal experience of being a pregnant mother on opioids, I am painfully aware of the stigma in healthcare associated with opioid use during pregnancy. Even as I write this, I can feel the sting of healthcare providers reading this who are thinking to themselves, "Oh…she's one of THOSE nurses…."

In my particular case, I injured my back through years of long-distance running. As a 25-year-old who was taking too much tramadol to get through the workday lifting nursing home patients, I was prescribed 90 mgs of morphine tabs per day. I had no idea at the time that this would become a lifelong problem. Luckily, I realized that opioids were affecting my life and personality in ways worse than the pain I felt before I started taking them. But the pain I experienced while trying to withdraw from them was far worse than both…withdrawal is a physical and psychological pain I had never known. I was so angry with myself, and I felt so weak. So, I sought out Suboxone and here I am, two children and 15 years later still taking this opioid.

Absolutely, the worst of the dismay and personal guilt felt over opioid use hits the hardest during pregnancy. Opioid-dependent pregnant patients are often advised to remain on opioids to lessen the risk of withdrawal and miscarriage, but I worried and guilted over it nonetheless. My first birth went smoothly, which lessened my fears. My second birth was very different, however; my son was born preterm and was admitted to the NICU. I asked a nurse if his agitation may be related to neonatal withdrawal and discovered none of the staff nor providers knew this had been an "opioid pregnancy" and that this baby…my baby…was a "drug baby." There was a noticeable, sudden shift in the demeanor and care of the NICU providers from that day forward. One nurse told me, "You have no idea what babies in withdrawal go through; it's beyond me how any mother can put them through that." To say her words felt like an absolute punch in the gut is an understatement, for there are no words to describe the sheer awfulness her words made me feel. Looking back, I wish I had the courage to stand up for myself, but I saw myself through her eyes as a "bad mom." There is nothing harder than being pregnant while on any medication that risks impact to your unborn child, but it is troubling that being a pregnant mother on opioid medication carries with it a heavier stigma than use of other medications, which often pose higher risks for newborns.

3 Conclusions and Future Directions

I hope these stories that are brought to the fore can be used by health systems and policymakers to be more responsive to the unique needs of vulnerable populations and, in particular, inform the construction of evidence-based interventions that mitigate disparities in accessing and navigating care for substance-using pregnant women who have largely been ignored in current substance use treatment and prevention.

The preliminary findings of this project point to the complicated journey of substance use treatment for pregnant women who are substance users. Barriers are not just a basic lack of insurance, and in many cases even if the women are insured, there are barriers to care that are informed by histories of experience with the healthcare system and historical and structural racism associated with institutions that provide care in Baltimore and legal and social structures that set the parameters of that care. Healthcare programs and social interventions need to be structured to account for the layers of clinical needs that come with substance use, including and especially mental healthcare needs and housing.

Acknowledgment The author would like to thank the many women and healthcare providers who provided invaluable insights through their perspective and experiences regarding improving care for substance-using pregnant women. The author would also like to acknowledge funding support from the Agency for Healthcare Research and Quality (AHRQ).

Glossary of Terms

Substance use The utilization and consumption of substances (with prescription or without prescription) or illicit substances that are associated with varying degrees of adverse maternal or fetal health. These include alcohol, tobacco, opioids, and other substances.

Criminalization The prohibition of substance use resulting in involvement of law enforcement or the state's legal and social services apparatus broadly.

Addiction According to the American Society of Addiction Medicine (ASAM), addiction is a treatable, chronic medical disease involving complex interactions among brain circuits, genetics, the environment, and an individual's life experiences. People with addiction use substances or engage in behaviors that become compulsive and often continue despite harmful consequences (ASAM).

Questions for Thought and Discussion

1. Define stigma. What are two specific ways stigma can reflect structural racism and inequalities at the societal level?
2. From the perspective of healthcare providers, do you feel that mandated reporting supports care for pregnant women who are substance users? Why or why not?

3. What are some barriers to care for pregnant women who are substance users? In what ways are these barriers unique to pregnant women compared to nonpregnant women?
4. How does racism play a role in preventing substance-using women from seeking care? How is racism embedded in institutions of care and our healthcare policies and practices?
5. In what ways does criminalizing substance use impact access to care and health outcomes? Be specific in identifying particular laws and policies that explicitly or by extension lead to criminalization.

References

Agency for Healthcare Research and Quality. *Increasing access to medication-assisted treatment of opioid abuse in rural primary care practices*. Rockville. Content last reviewed Feb 2017.

American Society of Addiction Medicine. *Definition of addiction*. https://www.asam.org/Quality-Science/definition-of-addiction. Accessed June 2020.

Angelotta, C., Weiss, C., Angelotta, J. W., et al. (2016). A moral or medical problem? The relationship between legal penalties and treatment practices for opioid use disorders in pregnant women. *Women's Health Issues, 26*(6), 595–601.

Beetham, T., Saloner, B., Wakeman, S. E., et al. (2019). Access to office-based buprenorphine treatment in areas with high rates of opioid-related mortality: An audit study. *Annals of Internal Medicine, 171*, 1–9.

Black Mamas Matter Alliance. *Advancing black maternal health*. https://blackmamasmatter.org. Accessed June 2020.

Centers for Disease Control (2019, November). *Racial and ethnic disparities continue in pregnancy-related deaths Black, American Indian/Alaska Native women most affected*. https://www.cdc.gov/media/releases/2019/p0905-racial-ethnic-disparities-pregnancy-deaths.html. Accessed Nov 2019.

Glaser, B. G. (1994). *More grounded theory methodology: A reader*. Mill Valley: Sociology Press.

Goffman, E. (1963). *Stigma: Notes on the management of spoiled identity*. New York: Simon & Schuster.

Harfeld, A., & Marlowe, K. (2017). Making America's children safe again: Advocating for CAPTA reform and beyond. *Juvenile and Family Court Journal, 68*(1), 115–128.

Health Policy Project. (2011). *Stigma and discrimination*. United States Agency for International Development (USAID).

Howarth, C. (2006). Race as stigma: Positioning the stigmatized as agents, not objects. *Journal of Community and Applied Social Psychology, 16*(6), 442–451. https://doi.org/10.1002/casp.898.

Krans, E. E., Kim, J. Y., James III, A. E., Kelley, D., & Jarlenski, M. P. (2019). Medication-assisted treatment use among pregnant women with opioid use disorder. *Obstetrics & Gynecology, 133*(5), 943–951.

National Advocates for Pregnant Women. Understanding CAPTA and State Obligations, September 2018. http://advocatesforpregnantwomen.org/CAPTA%20requirements%20for%20states_NAPW.pdf. Accessed 11 Oct 2019.

National Institute on Drug Abuse. (2019). National Institutes of Health; U.S. Department of Health and Human Services.

Paltrow, L. M., & Flavin, J. (2013). Arrests of and forced interventions on pregnant women in the United States, 1973–2005: Implications for women's legal status and public health. *Journal of Health Politics, Policy and Law, 38*(2), 299–343.

Parker, R., & Aggleton, P. (2003). HIV and AIDS-related stigma and discrimination: A conceptual framework and implications for action. *Social Science & Medicine, 57*(1), 13–24.

Saloner, B., & Karthikeyan, S. (2015). Changes in substance abuse treatment use among individuals with opioid use disorders in the United States, 2004-2013. *Journal of the American Medical Association, 314*(14), 1515–1517.

Saloner, B., & Lê Cook, B. (2013). Blacks and Hispanics are less likely than whites to complete addiction treatment, largely due to socioeconomic factors. *Health Affairs (Millwood), 32*(1), 135–145. https://doi.org/10.1377/hlthaff.2011.0983.

Stangl, A. L., Earnshaw, V. A., Logie, C. H., et al. (2019). The health stigma and discrimination framework: A global, crosscutting framework to inform research, intervention development, and policy on health-related stigmas. *BMC Medicine, 17*, 31. https://doi.org/10.1186/s12916-019-1271-3.

Stone, R. (2015). Pregnant women and substance use: fear, stigma, and barriers to care. *Health Justice, 3*, 2. Published 2015 February 12. https://doi.org/10.1186/s40352-015-0015-5.

Substance Abuse and Mental Health Services Administration (US). Office of the Surgeon General (US). (2016, November). Washington, DC: US Department of Health and Human Services.

Vedam, S., Stoll, K., Taiwo, T. K., et al. (2019). The giving voice to mothers study: Inequity and mistreatment during pregnancy and childbirth in the United States. *Reproductive Health, 16*, 77. https://doi.org/10.1186/s12978-019-0729-2.

Chapter 2
Protecting Workers from Opioid Misuse and Addiction

Jonathan Rosen

1 Introduction Background on the Public Health Crisis

The opioid crisis was declared a national public health emergency by the US Department of Health and Human Services on October 17, 2017 (HHS 2019a, b). The impact on the workplace is significant and certain occupations and industries are more highly affected, especially in industries with higher rates of occupational injury and illness. Effective workplace interventions are needed to prevent opioid misuse and addiction and to refer affected workers for treatment and recovery programs. Overcoming stigma and reforming punitive workplace substance abuse programs are fundamental to developing effective workplace intervention programs (Fig. 2.1).

Every day an estimated 130 people die from opioid-related drug overdoses. In 2017, 47,600 people died from opioid drug overdoses, 2.1 million people had an opioid misuse disorder, and 886,000 used heroin. More than 11 million people (4.2% of the population) misused prescription opioids (CDC 2019a, b). Only about 1 in 8 people (12.2%) who needed substance use disorder treatment received it in 2017 (SAMHSA 2018).

The CDC reports that life expectancy in the United States has declined for 3 years in a row (2014–2017) due to increased mortality related to drug overdoses (mainly opioids), suicide, and alcohol (NCHS 2017; TAH 2017). The decrease in life expectancy was paralleled by increased morbidity, including deteriorations in self-reported physical and mental health, and rising reports of chronic pain (Case and Deaton 2015).

J. Rosen (✉)
AJ Rosen & Associates LLC, Schenectady, NY, USA

J. M. Croff, J. Beaman (eds.), *Family Resilience and Recovery from Opioids and Other Addictions*, Emerging Issues in Family and Individual Resilience,
https://doi.org/10.1007/978-3-030-56958-7_2

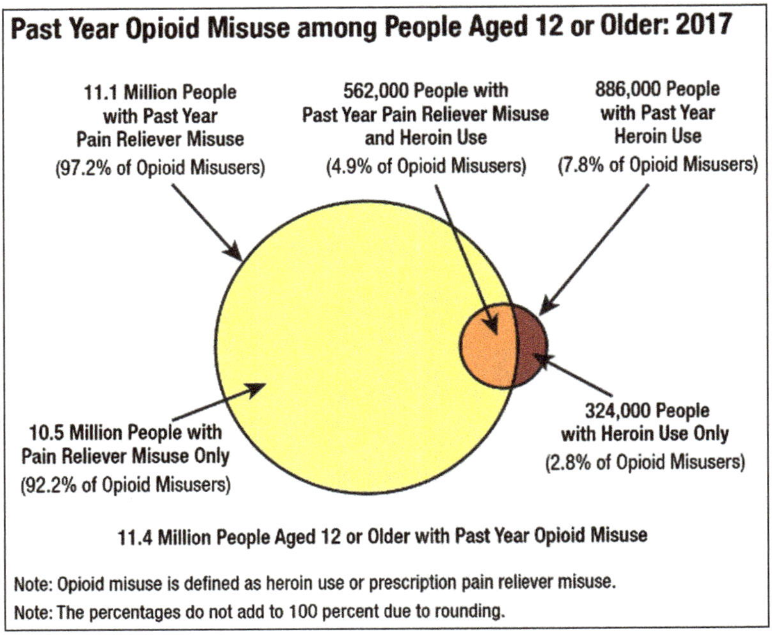

Fig. 2.1 SAMHSA key substance abuse and mental health indicators in the United States

1.1 Deaths of Despair

Several authors have reviewed the importance of social and economic disparities during the past 50 years and the impact of the resultant stress and hopelessness as a likely cause of the loss in life expectancy (Case and Deaton 2015). Increased inequality, poverty, de-industrialization, loss of union density, loss of pensions, frozen wages, temporary and contract work, and a hostile political environment are important occupational stressors that increase hopelessness and despair (Burris 2018). In a study in Allegheny County, Pennsylvania, case-level mortality data revealed an association between fatal overdose and poverty, with the highest fatality rates clustered in the region's deindustrialized communities. In interviews, workers who were in recovery described hopelessness and inadequate access to opportunity as driving factors for substance use (McLean 2016).

Other factors for substance use include work/life balance stress due to excessive use of mandatory overtime and nontraditional work schedules. According to one study, annual work hours are 4% higher than they were in 1980, amounting to an extra 1 h and 30 min at work per week. These extra hours at work mean less time with the family and reduce time available to play with children or help them with homework, as well as housework, sleep, recreation, and spousal and social activities (Dembe et al. 2005; Golden and Jorgens 2002). According to the Economic Policy Institute, "These sacrifices can translate into increased risk for accidents and injuries; greater chronic fatigue, stress, and related diseases; reduced parenting and family time; and diminished quality of goods and services" (EPI 2002).

Other impacts of job stress may include workplace bullying, harassment, violence, job burnout, and presenteeism. Presenteeism is when a worker is present at work when they should not be, such as when they have an illness or family problem (Hemp Paul 2004).

1.1.1 "Worst Man-Made Epidemic in Modern Medical History"[1]

In the mid-1990s, pharmaceutical companies reassured the medical community that patients would not become addicted to opioid pain relievers and healthcare providers began to prescribe them at greater rates (Hadland et al. 2019). Previously, opioids were mainly used for treating cancer-related pain and end-of-life palliative care. The pharmaceutical companies launched massive sales campaigns. Pain was declared the fifth vital sign and providers were pressured to increase their prescription of opioids. Providers wrote nearly a quarter of a billion opioid prescriptions in 2013, enough for every American adult to have their own bottle of pills. Purdue Pharma "pleaded guilty to misbranding OxyContin, a prescription opioid pain medication, with the intent to defraud or mislead" and paid a $600 million dollar settlement in 2007 in a federal lawsuit brought against it by the State of Virginia. Purdue Pharma generated over $30 billion from the sale of OxyContin since it was introduced (Van Zee 2009).

From the New York v. Purdue Pharma, 2018 summons,

> Purdue spent over $1 billion on a sales and marketing blitz, unprecedented in the history of controlled substances, which targeted doctors in multiple subspecialties, nurses, physicians' assistants, patients, advocacy groups, accreditation organizations, regulators, and others. (New York v. Purdue Pharma 2018)

Increased prescriptions led to widespread misuse of both prescription and nonprescription opioids before it became clear that these medications could indeed be highly addictive (Van Zee 2009). Gary Franklin, MD, Medical Director for the Washington State Workers' Compensation system, refers to the crisis as the "worst man-made epidemic in modern medical history." More than 200,000 people died from prescription opioids between 1999 and 2016 (CDC 2020a, b). More than 191 million opioid prescriptions were dispensed to American patients in 2017—with wide variation across states (CDC 2020a, b).

Purdue Pharma's sales force engaged in a new form of marketing directly to primary care doctors, distributing 340,000 free samples, in addition to gifts, trips,

[1] Quote from Gary Franklin, MD, research Professor in the Department of Environmental and Occupational Health Sciences and in the Department of Medicine at the University of Washington (UW) and Medical Director of the Washington State Department of Labor and Industries (L&I) from 1988 to the present, and has more than a 25-year history of developing and administering workers' compensation health care policy and conducting outcomes research.

and educational credits to providers (Van Zee 2009). The extensive sales force was paid $60 million in bonuses (Van Zee 2009).

1.2 Cost of the Opioid Crisis

The estimated total economic cost of the opioid crisis in 2015 was $504 billion, accounting for 2.8% of gross domestic product (Council of Economic Advisers 2017). Opioid use among workers can impact workplace safety and health, productivity, and increase use of sick leave and healthcare benefits. Lost productivity related to nonfatal overdoses and incarceration accounted for $20 billion, while fatal overdoses cost $21.5 billion in lost productivity and healthcare costs (O'Neill Hayes and Manos 2018). Nearly one million people were out of the workforce due to the opioid crisis. An estimated 66.2% of self-reported illicit opioid users were employed full or part time (SAMHSA 2016).

1.3 Determining Work Relatedness

In 2002, Dr. Franklin and colleagues discovered that injured workers in Washington State were dying from prescription opioid overdoses in increasing numbers. Incredibly, many of these cases involved back injuries or carpal tunnel syndrome. Subsequently, Washington State developed guidelines, regulations, and provider education that have led to a reduced death toll. Deaths declined 27% from 2008 to 2012 due to these interventions (Franklin et al. 2015). Additional studies by Dr. Franklin and colleagues have revealed that opioid prescribing in Washington's Workers' Compensation system failed to reduce pain or help injured workers return to work (Franklin et al. 2008; Webster et al. 2007).

1.3.1 Massachusetts Department of Public Health Study

The Massachusetts Department of Public Health published a report in August 2018 on opioid deaths by industry and occupation that revealed 4302 deaths in the 4-year period of 2011–2015 (MA DPH 2018). Construction and extraction workers had a 6 times greater rate of death than the average for all Massachusetts workers. Twenty-four percent of the deaths were in construction and extraction alone. Workers in the farming, fishing, and forestry had a rate 5 times the average. The study concluded that industries with high rates of occupational injury had high rates of opioid fatality. The rate was also higher in occupations with lower availability of paid sick leave and job security.

This study did not determine how many of the cases derived directly from a work-related injury or illness; however, that research is ongoing. The study recommended addressing the following key educational and policy interventions (Fig. 2.2):

- Workplace hazards that cause injuries for which opioids are prescribed
- Appropriate pain management following injury, including safer opioid prescribing
- Access to evidence-based treatment for opioid use disorders
- Overdose prevention education (MA DPH 2018)

1.3.2 National Institute for Occupational Safety and Health (NIOSH) Study

In August 2018, NIOSH published "Occupational patterns in opioid-involved overdose Deaths—United States, 2007–2012" evaluating data from 26 occupational groups from 21 states (Hardaur Morano et al. 2018). They identified 57,810 drug overdose deaths from 26 occupational groups and found that rates were highest in six groups: (1) construction, (2) extraction, (3) food preparation and serving, (4) healthcare and technical, (5) healthcare support, and (6) personal care and service.

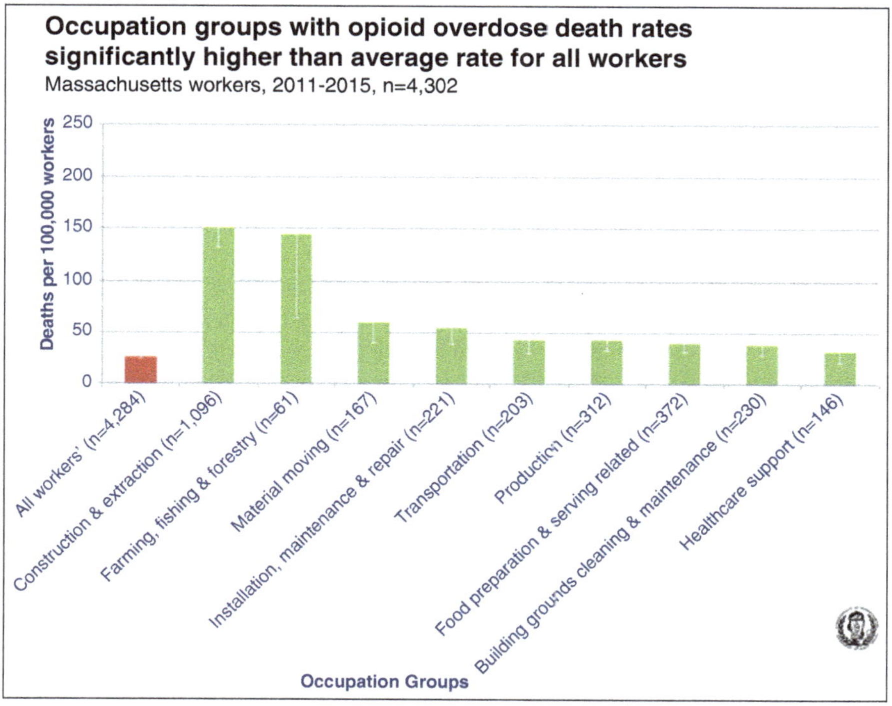

Fig. 2.2 From Mass Department of Public Health Report (MA DPH 2018)

The study revealed 7402 (13% of the total) drug overdose deaths among construction workers alone.

The authors suggested the following examples of programs that might address both licit and illicit opioid use:

- Comprehensive drug-free workplace programs
- Employee assistance programs
- Peer-support networks
- Education targeted to employees and employers
- Continued evaluation of the effectiveness and impact of these programs and interventions as needed to prevent opioid misuse and abuse and to reduce opioid-related morbidity and mortality

1.3.3 Reported Work-Related Injuries, Illnesses, and Fatalities

In 2017, private employers reported 2.8 million work injuries and illnesses and 5147 occupational fatalities to the US Bureau of Labor Statistics (US Bureau of Labor Statistics 2018a, b). Overdoses due to nonmedical use of drugs or alcohol while at work increased 25% from 217 in 2016 to 272 in 2017. This was the fifth consecutive year in which workplace overdose deaths increased by at least 25% (US Bureau of Labor Statistics 2018a, b).

A Government Accounting Office report and other studies have addressed the significant underreporting of occupational injuries and illnesses to the Bureau of Labor Statistics. Underreporting is due to a number of factors such as fear of retaliation, post-accident drug testing, incentive reward programs, and in effort to keep workers' compensation costs down (GAO 2009). In one study it was determined that only 25% of severe injuries among Hispanics and 60% among white workers in small construction companies had been recorded (Dong et al. 2011).

Studies have also documented that many injured workers do not file workers' compensation (WC) claims. One study documented that 55–79% of people who could qualify for WC never file a claim (Fan et al. 2006). Using capture–recapture analysis of work-related musculoskeletal disorders (MSDs) in Connecticut, Morse estimated that only 5.5–7.9% of MSD cases appear to have been reported to WC annually (Fan Bonauto et al. 2006). Although it has not been determined how many of the opioid deaths documented in the Massachusetts and NIOSH studies began as treatment for work injuries and related pain, it is understood that physical and emotional pain are pathways to opioid misuse, addiction, and death (Franklin et al. 2008; Massachusetts DPHs 2018; NIOSH 2019). Delays in getting diagnostic or treatment approvals from the healthcare or workers' compensation insurance systems may also contribute to this conundrum.

1.4 Applying the Public Health and Industrial Hygiene Approach to Prevention

The public health model includes primary, secondary, and tertiary approaches to prevention (CDC 2019a, b). Primary prevention features interventions designed to prevent exposure from occurring. Secondary prevention occurs during the early stages of disease before onset of signs and symptoms. Tertiary prevention includes methods that aim to ameliorate the impact of disease once it has been established (CDC 2019a, b). Application of the public health model for prevention of opioid misuse is detailed in the chart below (Fig. 2.3).

1.4.1 Primary Prevention

The goal of primary prevention is to avoid injury and illness through effective safety and health programs. Effective prevention of occupational injury and exposures will result in fewer workers needing medical care that includes pain treatment, a potential pathway to opioid misuse and addiction (CDC 2019a, b).

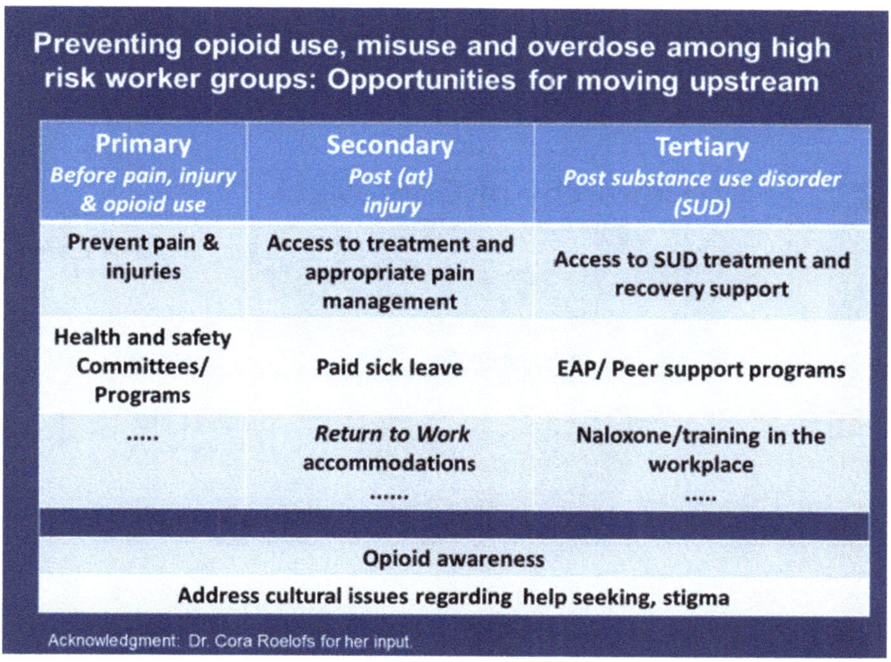

Fig. 2.3 Davis, L, Massachusetts DPHm 2019. EAP = Employee Assistance Program

A key step is for employers, unions, and other workplace stakeholders to evaluate the risk factors for workplace injury and illnesses by looking at available data sources such as OSHA 300 logs and workers' compensation records. Other methods for assessing workplace hazards include interviews of injured workers, focus groups, and worker surveys. The point of these assessments is to identify the root cause of injuries and exposures by looking at the work environment, equipment, and documenting safety and health hazards. Once the hazards are identified, efforts shift to hazard control using the hierarchy of control measures which is recognized as the appropriate approach (Fig. 2.4).

According to NIOSH,

> The idea behind this hierarchy is that the control methods at the top of graphic are potentially more effective and protective than those at the bottom. Following this hierarchy normally leads to the implementation of inherently safer systems, where the risk of illness or injury has been substantially reduced. (NIOSH 2019)

The hierarchy may be applied in the following manner when considering selection of hazard controls:

- Elimination: Can a process be automated, or can a step be eliminated so that a hazard is removed?
- Substitution: Can a hazardous material, chemical, or process be substituted for a less hazardous material, chemical, or process?
- Engineering controls: Can a machine, mechanism, or device be engineered with a safer design?

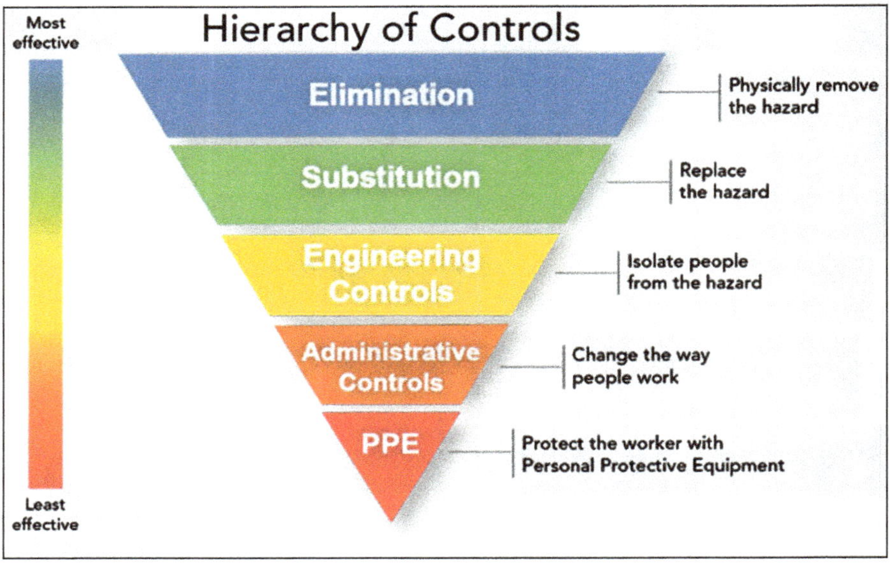

Fig. 2.4 NIOSH Hierarchy of Controls, https://www.cdc.gov/niosh/topics/hierarchy/default.html

- Administrative and work practice controls: If none of the above can be achieved or if risk still exists after the hierarchy has been implemented, can a worker interact with a process or procedure in a safer manner that may involve training and education? Might the culture and climate of institutional safety improve outcomes? Might alternating tasks and/or shifts improve outcomes?
- PPE: If none of the above isolate or remove the hazard, only then shall PPE be used. Is there PPE that could further reduce a hazard, including eye protection, gloves, protective clothing, etc.? Is it readily accessible wherever it is needed, immediately at the time it is needed?

Utilizing the hierarchy to assess risk and build preventive programs and controls is an essential approach for preventing injury and illness.

1.4.2 Ergonomics

NIOSH defines it as "the science of fitting workplace conditions and job demands to the capabilities of the working population" (NIOSH 2019). When jobs are not designed to accommodate people's physical attributes and differences, the result can be musculoskeletal disorders (MSDs). MSDs affect the muscles, nerves, blood vessels, ligaments, and tendons (NIOSH 2019). Workers in many different industries and occupations are exposed to risk factors for MSDs that include lifting, bending, reaching, pushing, and pulling, moving heavy loads, working in awkward body postures, and performing repetitive tasks (NIOSH 2019) (Fig. 2.5).

In 2017 there were 344,970 MSD cases reported to the US Bureau of Labor Statistics, and they comprised 34% of the lost work time cases in manufacturing alone (BLS 2018a, b). The average number of lost work days was 12, compared to 8 for other work-related injuries. Musculoskeletal disorders are the single largest cause of work-related illness, accounting for over 33% of all newly reported occupational illnesses in the general population and approximately 77% in construction workers (Gopireddy et al. 2016). This type of injury is also associated with widespread use of prescription pain medication as previously noted.

Fig. 2.5 Examples of MSDs

Examples of Musculoskeletal Disorders (MSDs)

- Carpal tunnel syndrome
- Tendinitis
- Rotator cuff injuries (affects the shoulder)
- Epicondylitis (affects the elbow)
- Trigger finger
- Muscle strains and low back injuries

Workplace stress and the organization of work are additional risk factors. For example, construction workers typically do not get paid when they are not working, and they frequently work long hours doing physically demanding work. The norm is for construction workers to work hard when the opportunity arises including 12- to 16-h days and 6- to 7-day work weeks. This results in many working in constant pain. The impact of prescription opioids used for pain treatment or self-medication is clear as the construction industry has the highest rate of opioid fatalities. Ergonomic solutions are clearly an important preventive intervention. Paid time off, for sickness and vacation, is another reform that would address the underlying stressors.

Examples of ergonomic interventions include safe patient handling programs in healthcare that have proven to reduce back injuries that are epidemic among nurses and nurses' aides. These programs have been proven to be cost effective while reducing workers' compensation and related costs (Siddharthan et al. 2005). In one study the introduction of a safe handling program in 9 hospitals reduced injuries by 71% and lost workdays by 90% (OSHA 2013) (Fig. 2.6).

Two examples of ergonomic solutions in construction are illustrated below (NIOSH XE "NIOSH" 2007). These are examples of engineering controls used for preventing MSDs as described previously in the hierarchy of controls (Fig. 2.7).

After decades of research, hearings, and debate in November 2000, the Occupational Safety and Health Administration (OSHA) issued an enforceable ergonomics standard to prevent MSDs. It was rescinded by Congress within 4 months under the Congressional Review Act, prohibiting OSHA from ever issuing a substantially similar standard (Delp et al. 2014). This dilemma has enabled the epidemic of sprains and strains to continue unabated, as employers are not required

Key elements of an ergonomics program include:

1. Provide Management Commitment and support.
2. Involve Workers - A participatory ergonomic approach, where workers:
   a. Identify and provide information about hazards in their workplaces.
   b. Voice concerns and suggestions for reducing exposure to risk factors and by evaluating ergonomic improvements.
3. Provide Training
4. Identify Problems - identify and assess ergonomic problems in the workplace before they result in MSDs.
5. Encourage Early Reporting of MSD Symptoms - Early reporting can accelerate the job assessment and improvement process, helping to prevent or reduce the progression of symptoms, the development of serious injuries, and subsequent lost-time claims.
6. Implement Solutions to Control Hazards.
7. Evaluate Progress

Fig. 2.6 Key elements of an ergonomics program (OSHA 2020)

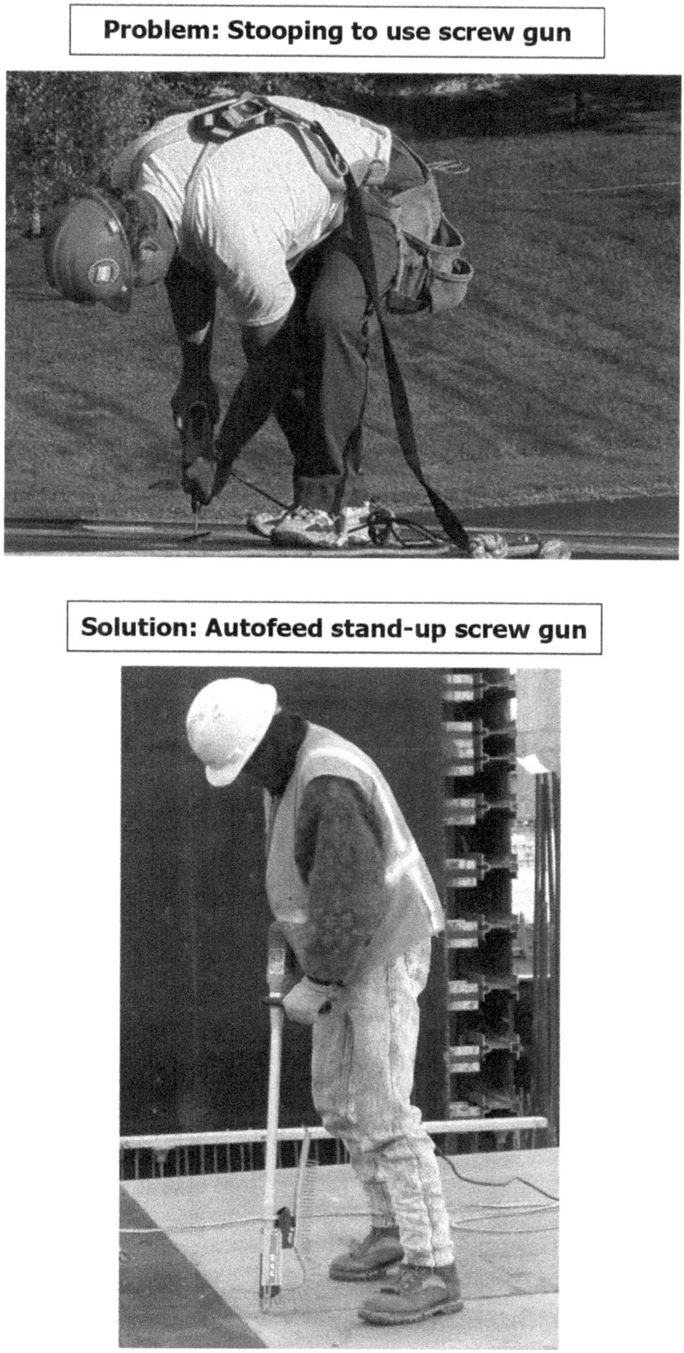
Problem: Stooping to use screw gun
Solution: Autofeed stand-up screw gun

Fig. 2.7 Example of ergonomic solutions (NIOSH 2007)

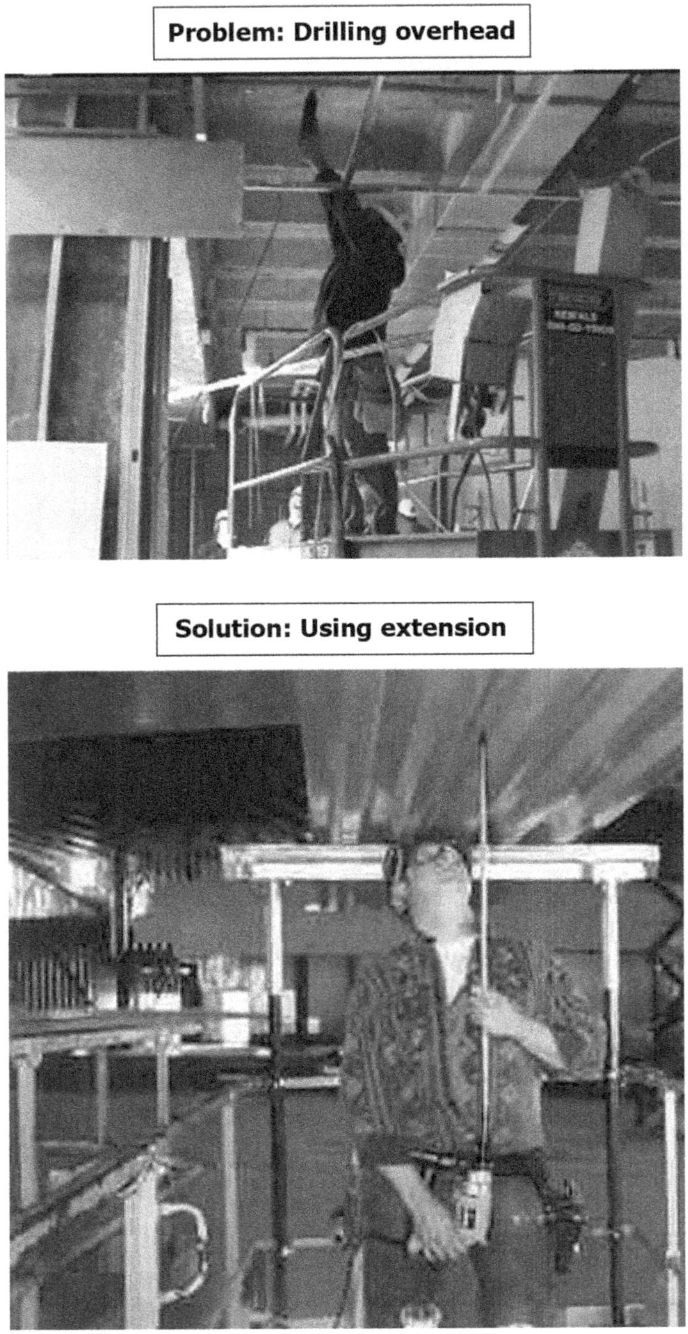

Fig. 2.7 (continued)

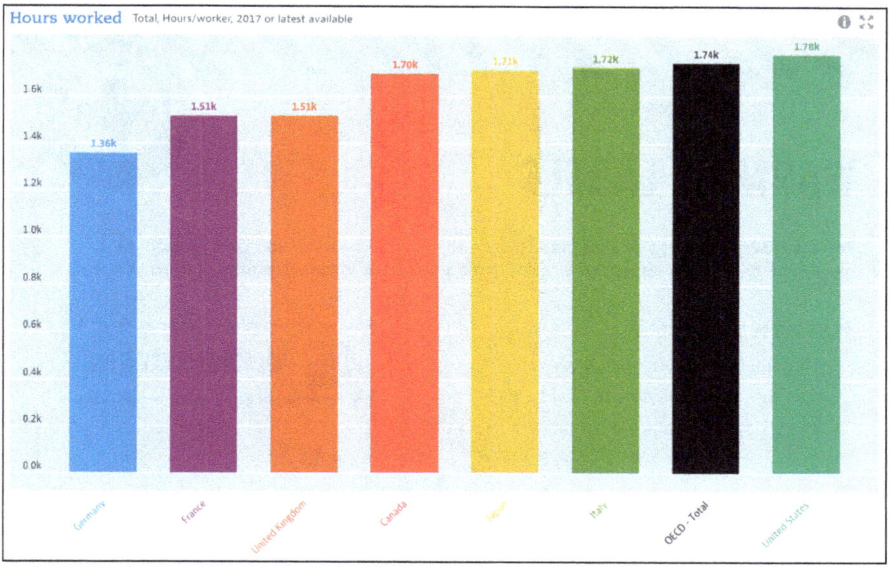

Fig. 2.8 Total average hours worked per year by country

to evaluate and control ergonomic risks except in 11 states that have passed safe patient handling laws applicable only to healthcare facilities (Weinmeyer 2016).

There are many other occupational hazards that cause pain and potential misuse of opioids. In response to the opioid crisis, every effected place of employment should review their evaluation of job hazards and safety and health management systems.

1.4.3 Occupational Stress

Construction workers are not the only occupation that work long hours doing physically demanding work. According to NIOSH, annual work hours have steadily increased over several decades in the United States and have surpassed that of Japan and Western Europe (Caruso et al. 2004; OECD 2017). The NIOSH analysis showed a pattern of deteriorating performance on "psychophysiological tests as well as injuries while working long hours was observed across study findings, particularly with very long shifts and when 12-hour shifts combined with more than 40 h of work a week" (Caruso et al. 2004; OECD 2019, iv). Two studies comparing 8- and 12-h shifts reported higher rates of fatigue, alcohol, and tobacco use (Caruso et al. 2004) (Fig. 2.8).

The healthcare industry has adopted a grueling 12-hour shift for direct care staff, and due to nursing shortages, it is common for nurses to work double shifts. Lipscomb et al. (2002) found that 12-hour shifts and 40 or more hours of work per week were associated with elevated risk for neck, shoulder, and back disorders as

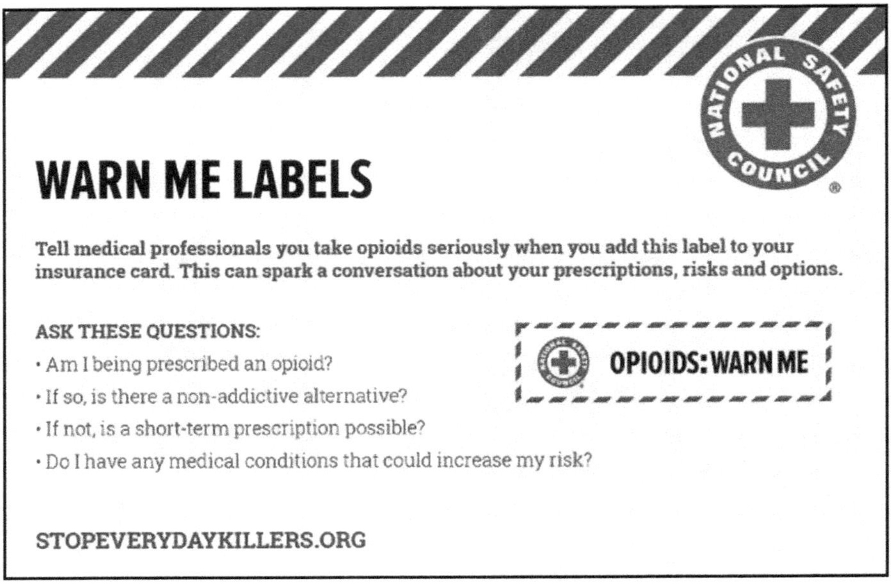

Fig. 2.9 Warn Me labels

compared to five 8-h shifts per week (Lipscomb et al. 2002). This study also documented that these shifts were associated with increased rates of MSDs among nurses.

There are many other industries with high rates of mandatory overtime, extended hours, and split shifts including transportation and manufacturing. Work organization factors can give rise to work/family conflict, fatigue, disruption to sleep cycles, and heighten the risk of occupational injury as well as negative psychological effects.

1.4.4 Secondary Prevention

A recommended step in preventing misuse of opioids is the development of an organizational process such as a subcommittee within an organization's Safety and Health or Labor/Management Committee to develop training and awareness of opioid misuse and addiction (Fig. 2.9).

A committee should be multidisciplinary and involve relevant workplace stakeholders including frontline workers who have direct knowledge of workplace hazards, stressors, and culture. Providing training on avoidance of the misuse of opioids and assistance to injured workers is an important intervention to prepare workers in the event they become injured at work or at home (Fig. 2.10).

The development of tools to assist injured workers in interacting with healthcare providers should include materials such as:

- Language appropriate fact sheets that explain opioid associated risks
- Checklists with questions to discuss with healthcare providers about opioid prescribing and alternative pain treatments

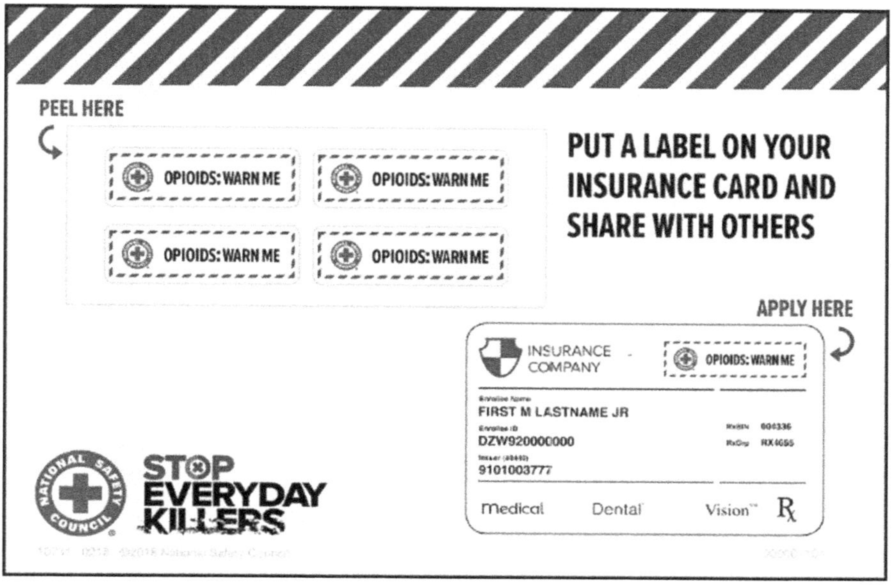

Fig. 2.10 Put a Warn Me label on your insurance card

- Warn Me labels and stickers that can be placed on health insurance cards, "Opioids: Warn Me" (available from the National Safety Council at http://safety.nsc.org/stop-everyday-killers-supplies)
- Stericycle Seal&Send Envelope is used to get rid of controlled substances for destruction (available from the National Safety Council at http://safety.nsc.org/stop-everyday-killers-supplies)
- Information on safe storage and disposal of narcotics at home

1.4.5 Tertiary Prevention

Tertiary prevention focuses on access to treatment and recovery programs in the workplace for workers who need such support (Fig. 2.11).

According to the National Safety Council, 70% of employers feel that prescription drugs have impacted them, but 76% do not offer training, 81% lack a comprehensive policy for substance abuse in the workplace, and just 41% who perform drug tests do test for synthetic opioids (Hersman 2017). An additional concern is whether employer insurance benefits are adequate at providing alternative pain therapies and coverage for mental health and/or substance abuse treatment.

An Ohio survey of 4713 (3229 business organizations and 1484 community leaders) conducted by the Drug-Free Workforce Community Initiative found the following (Working Partners Drug-Free Workforce Community Initiative 2017):

- Only about half of surveyed workplaces have a significant written substance abuse policy, more than one page.

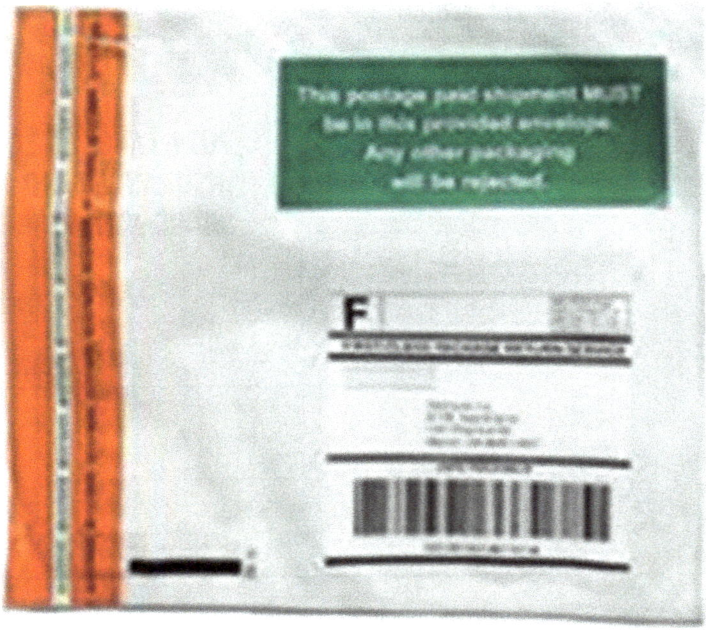

Fig. 2.11 Prepaid drug disposal mailer

- Only about 26.4% of businesses conduct annual drug-free workplace employee education.
- Even fewer businesses, 23.7%, conduct annual supervisor training.
- Most businesses, 61%, currently drug test. This number is even higher, 78.3%, when we remove workplaces with fewer than 25 employees.
- Nearly half of businesses do not know what narcotics are being tested.
- Less than half of the businesses, 45.2%, believe treatment works for substance abuse problems.
- Only 1 in 12 employers would consider hiring an applicant who tested positive, then came back later after testing negative and being cleared by a counselor.
- Disciplinary action for current employees who test positive varies from providing a second chance, termination, or action decided on a case-by-case basis.
    - 26.8% terminate
    - 31% second chance
    - 25.2% decide on a case-by-case basis
    - 17% other
- 40% of businesses do not have or don't know if they have a professional resource identified when an employee needs help with a drug and/or alcohol problem (Breakout Box 2.1).

Breakout Box 2.1. Focus on Practice

Currently, I am the director of workforce development for an industrial park. In this role, we're really kind of working on behalf of the tenants at the industrial park, where we have just under 80 companies, and approximately 4500 full-time employees working for the individual companies throughout the park. At this time, we have pre-employment drug testing and then we test only for cause. We have a policy as an organization, but we are not involved in the individual policy making for the companies that exist within the park. However, our organizations and partners provide employee education by doing a lot of lunch and learn regarding the drug issue. A lot of that has been with the new marijuana laws. And so, but obviously some of that also delves into the opiates. The sessions are not separate from the supervisors; they do lunch and learn events together. We do offer an EAP, employee assistance program, so that people who have encountered addiction in some sort of way could seek help at work for counseling or services, but again, you know, we are fairly small. Our total employees are approximately 30. We've got an administration arm and park maintenance arm and then also own and operate the water treatment facility. So, the EAP is in place with our organization, but I'm also aware that other organizations and other businesses in the park also have policies of their own.

– Scott Fry, Director of Workforce Development

1.5 History of Punitive Workplace Substance Abuse Policies

A major obstacle to workers coming forward to discuss substance abuse or underlying mental health problems are punitive workplace substance abuse policies. In workplaces with zero tolerance policies, a positive drug test leads to termination of employment. Last chance agreements also imply that workers will only get one opportunity for treatment and recovery, even though it is recognized that opioid use disorder is a "chronic, relapsing disorder characterized by compulsive drug seeking and use despite adverse consequences" (National Institute on Drug Abuse 2019). Some policies allow for two or three chances at treatment before a worker is terminated. Although these policies are more supportive than zero tolerance or last chance agreements, they still do not recognize that it is the nature of opioid use disorder that it often takes multiple attempts at treatment before a person remains in recovery. Punitive policies beg the question why a worker would voluntarily come forward for help if they know that it could lead to a loss of employment.

Opioid use disorder is recognized as a disease by the Centers for Disease Control, the American Medical Association, and the American Society of Addiction Medicine. Criteria for diagnosis of opioid use disorder (OUD) are contained in the Diagnostic and Statistical Manual of Mental Disorders (DSM–5). However, due to stigma and punitive policies, OUD is usually treated differently than other diseases by employers. In comparison, it would be considered outrageous if a worker had cancer and an employer offered them a last chance agreement if the cancer came back.

The history of the punitive approach dates to 1981 when an aircraft crashed aboard the USS Nimitz, an American aircraft carrier and one of the largest war ships in the world, killing 14 people, injuring 48, and resulting in an estimated cost of $150 million (Connecticut Department of Public Health 2018). It was discovered that drug use by the military personnel on the plane was a contributing factor to the disaster (Connecticut Department of Public Health 2018). Prior to this event, the military typically provided substance abuse treatment and only began a more punitive approach after the accident (Connecticut Department of Public Health 2018). After the accident, the Department of Defense employed a zero-tolerance policy and authorized punitive actions including court martial and discharge to be used against service members who failed drug tests (Connecticut Department of Public Health 2018).

In 1986, the drug-free workplace and zero-tolerance policy was expanded to the entire federal government workforce through Executive Order 12564.46 (Connecticut Department of Public Health 2018). In 1988, Congress expanded the drug-free workplace concept and zero-tolerance policy into the private sector by passing the Drug-Free Workplace Act, still in effect today, which requires government contractors to establish a drug-free workplace policy and penalize any violating employees (Connecticut Department of Public Health 2018).

1.5.1 The War on Drugs

In 1968, President Nixon initiated “the war on drugs” criminalizing addiction, installing punitive measures against drug users, and increasing incarceration (Moore and Elkavich 2008). All presidents that followed have embraced the war on drugs which has greatly expanded courts, prisons, and jails but had little to no effect on the use of drugs (Moore and Elkavich 2008). Urban communities of color have been hardest hit (Moore and Elkavich 2008). Between 1972 and 2008, there was a five-fold increase in incarceration without a comparable drop in drug use or crime (Moore and Elkavich 2008).

African Americans are incarcerated in state prisons across the country at more than five times the rate of whites, and at least ten times the rate in five states. Persons of color compose 60% of the incarcerated population. In 1996, Blacks constituted 62.6% of drug offenders in state prisons. Nationwide, the rate of persons admitted to prison on drug charges for Black men is 13 times that for White men, and in 10 states, the rates are 26 to 57 times those for White men. People of color are not more likely to do drugs; Black men do not have an abnormal predilection for intoxication. They are, however, more likely to be arrested and prosecuted for their use (Moore and Elkavich 2008; Lassiter 2015; SAMHSA 2014).

The bottom line is that the war on drugs has failed to reduce the demand for and use of drugs. That must be dealt with by dealing with the stressors in the workplace and in society that are driving the crisis.

1.6 Putting Programs in Place to Reduce Stigma in the Workplace

Shaming and disgracing people with mental health or substance abuse problems is a major deterrent to them coming forward in the workplace for help. The combined impact of punitive workplace substance abuse policies and stigma are very effective at keeping people who need help from talking to workplace leaders, union officials, and coworkers. The workplace climate should encourage workers who are suffering from chronic stress, workplace injury, or substance abuse to feel comfortable talking about these issues, without fear of reprisal or discrimination.

Employee assistance programs (EAPs) have been widely established across industries since the 1970s. However, there is marked difference in utilization and effectiveness (Weiss 2010). Some are internal models where staff are hired or personnel are trained to be available to talk to workers who are experiencing a broad spectrum of personnel problems. Typically, the EAP serves as a referral source. The external model typically involves access to a contractor who provides either direct support or referral services.

Some of the major concerns are whether workers trust the confidentiality of the EAP program and if workplace policies and culture act as a deterrent to workers using EAP services (Delaney et al. 1998). An additional obstacle is when employer provided health benefits that are not adequate in covering mental health and substance abuse treatment. Another feature of EAPs is that workers must initiate services. The EAP personnel are forbidden from proactively approaching workers, even if they know they need help.

Employers, unions, and other workplace stakeholders should review the design and utilization of EAP programs to ensure they are effective and accessible. Stigma and fear are significant obstacles, preventing workers who need substance abuse or mental health counseling from coming forward and accessing available services. Open communication about these uncomfortable topics and moving to nonpunitive programs can help create an environment where effected workers are more likely to access treatment.

1.6.1 Peer Support Programs

Development of peer support is fundamental to breaking down barriers. One example is the International Union of Operating Engineers Local 478's (Hamden, Ct) Member Assistance Program (MAP) (Zimmer 2018). This construction union established its MAP to address opioid and alcohol addiction, suicide, and behavioral health in the workplace. They have the cooperation of 248 out of 250 contractors with which they have collective bargaining agreements. This program extends the definition of peer from a person in recovery to a person in recovery from the same union or work organization. This model allows for more proactive support and takes advantage of peer relationships established through working together over time.

In this MAP, the union has established relationships with treatment providers and has been able to get members into treatment in a variety of programs within 12 h. Additionally, the union has hired two certified mental health/substance abuse counselors who provide support and leadership to the program. Every Thursday they hold peer support meetings at the union hall that are open to family members and nonunion construction workers. They report that 80% of those who entered the program and went into treatment for substance use disorder did not relapse. A key is that the peers are available 24/7 to support one another's recovery and together provide an alternative lifestyle. The union is also working on providing a peer advocacy certification training program to enhance the impact of this peer network.

1.7 Model Nonpunitive Workplace Substance Abuse Program

Alternatives to discipline programs have been available for decades, especially in healthcare where more than 40 Boards of Nursing have such programs (Cadiz et al. 2015; Monroe et al. 2013; SPAN New York State 2017). Rather than terminating the employee and rescinding their professional license, the employee signs a consent agreement to enter substance abuse treatment, temporarily suspends their professional license, participates in an individualized recovery program, agrees to periodic drug testing, and has limited access to narcotics for a period of 2–5 years. These programs vary by state and institution. However, research shows where they are least punitive; they have been very successful in helping nurses with substance use disorder recover and return to work. These programs are also designed to protect patient well-being by removing impaired healthcare workers from the care setting (Bettinardi-Angres et al. 2012) (Fig. 2.12).

Key elements of a nonpunitive workplace drug program are outlined in the graphic to the right. They include the incorporation of written policies that are based in employee involvement and feedback, training, access to adequate treatment programs, and implementation of alternate duty assignments and leave without fear of punitive action (Fig. 2.13).

1.8 Conclusion

The bottom line is understanding that opioid use disorder is a disease and not primarily a criminal or disciplinary matter. Preventive efforts begin with addressing workplace hazards and stressors. Developing training and nonpunitive workplace programs is key.

Work is healthy; it gives people a sense of purpose and structure and puts money in their pockets. Work directly improves the economic viability and sustainability of communities.

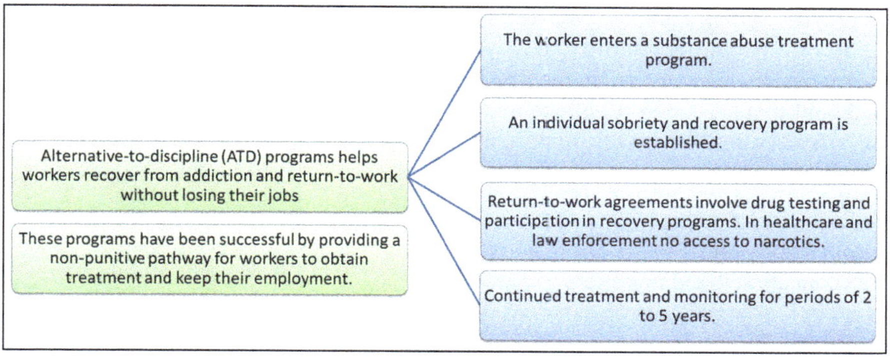

Fig. 2.12 Alternative-to-discipline programs

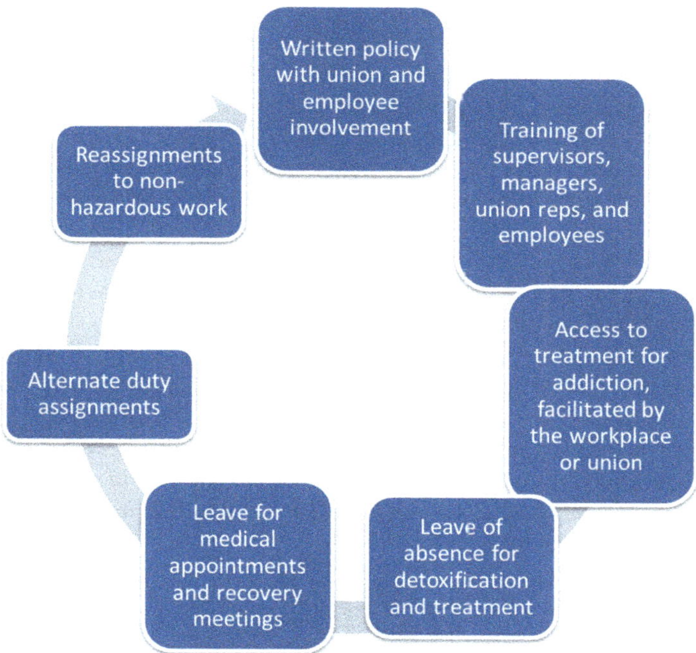
Written policy with union and employee involvement
Training of supervisors, managers, union reps, and employees
Access to treatment for addiction, facilitated by the workplace or union
Leave of absence for detoxification and treatment
Leave for medical appointments and recovery meetings
Alternate duty assignments
Reassignments to non-hazardous work

Fig. 2.13 Model workplace drug program

Investing in prevention and a renewed approach to workplace mental health and drug programs will undoubtedly save lives and help to rehumanize the workplace. In early 2019, the US Department of Labor announced that it is providing 22 million dollars to six states alone in National Health Emergency (NHE) Dislocated Worker Demonstration Grants to train people in recovery and provide incentives to employers to hire them. Several states are also providing tax incentives for employers to hire people in recovery. But why should employers fire workers with substance use disorder disease in the first place? Rather, employers should reform their drug and mental health programs and put an end to this revolving door. This will help their bottom line while simultaneously assisting workers, their families, and the communities in which they live reestablish healthy, productive, and meaningful lives.

Implications and Future Directions
Key educational and policy interventions:

1. As a means of primary prevention, hazards causing injuries must be evaluated and addressed using the hierarchy of controls. Interventions and controls should be developed that aim to strengthen programs to identify and mitigate workplace hazards that cause injuries for which opioids are prescribed.
2. Workplace education and training about opioid misuse, addiction, and mental health should be provided to workers, supervisors, union officials, and managers.
3. Workplace initiatives should educate injured workers and provide them with tools such as checklists they can use with healthcare providers to discuss appropriate pain management following injury, alternative pain management strategies, and safer opioid prescribing.
4. Develop worksite strategies to address stigma and demonization of workers who have mental health or substance use disorders and create nonpunitive drug policies where workers can talk about these issues and seek help without fear of reprisals.
5. Employers, labor unions, and other workplace stakeholders should develop and strengthen programs such as employee assistance, member assistance, and peer advocacy designed to encourage workers with mental health or substance use problems to come forward and connect with treatment and recovery resources.
6. Employers should ensure that coverage for mental health and substance use disorder treatment is adequate to provide workers with the support that is needed.
7. Continued evaluation of the effectiveness and impact of these programs and interventions are needed to prevent opioid misuse and to reduce opioid-related morbidity and mortality.

Acknowledgment I would like to express my heartfelt thanks to Amber Mitchell, Dr.PH., M.P.H., C.P.H., Executive Director, International Safety Center, for her helpful review and editing of the chapter.

Glossary of Terms

Addiction Opioid addiction is defined as a chronic, relapsing disorder characterized by compulsive drug seeking and use despite adverse consequences. It is considered a brain disorder, because it involves functional changes to brain circuits involved in reward, stress, and self-control, and those changes may last a long time after a person has stopped taking drugs.

Bureau of Labor Statistics (BLS) BLS is a unit of the US Department of Labor. It is the principal fact-finding agency for the US government in the broad field of labor economics and statistics and serves as a principal agency of the US Federal Statistical System.

Carpal tunnel syndrome Carpal tunnel syndrome is a condition that causes numbness, tingling and other symptoms in the hand and arm. Carpal tunnel syndrome is caused by a compressed nerve in the carpal tunnel, a narrow passageway on the palm side of your wrist.

Centers for Disease Control and Prevention (CDC) CDC is part of the federal Health and Human Services Agency. CDC works to protect America from health, safety, and security threats, both foreign and in the United States. Whether diseases start at home or abroad, are chronic or acute, are curable or preventable, or are caused by human error or deliberate attack, CDC fights disease and supports communities and citizens to do the same.

Dependence Dependence occurs when users become susceptible to withdrawal symptoms. Withdrawal symptoms occur only in patients who have developed tolerance.

Employee assistance programs (EAP) An EAP is a confidential work-based intervention program designed to assist employees in resolving personal problems that may be adversely affecting them. EAPs assist workers with issues like alcohol or substance use disorder as well as a broad range of issues such as child or elder care, relationship challenges, financial or legal problems, wellness matters, and traumatic events like workplace violence. EAPs may be internal or external and typically refer to users rather than providing direct counseling.

Ergonomics Ergonomics is the science of fitting the job to the worker. Workstations and tools are designed to reduce work-related musculoskeletal disorders. Work-related risk factors include lifting, bending, reaching, pushing, pulling, moving heavy loads, working in awkward body postures, and performing repetitive tasks.

Fentanyl Fentanyl is a powerful synthetic opioid that is similar to morphine but is 50 to 100 times more potent. It is a prescription drug that is also made and used illegally. Like morphine, it is a medicine that is typically used to treat patients with severe pain.

Government Accounting Office (GAO) The GAO is a federal agency that monitors and audits government spending and operations. The GAO tracks how the legislative and executive branches of the government use taxpayer dollars and then provides results directly to Congress.

Hierarchy of controls The hierarchy of controls is the accepted method in the field of occupational safety health for selecting corrective measures to prevent occupational exposures, injuries, and illnesses. The hierarchy starts with the most effective approach and the least effective is at the bottom as follows: elimination, substitution, engineering controls, administrative controls, and personal protective equipment.

Industry Any general business activity, commercial or public enterprise, for example, automobile industry or healthcare industry.

Job burnout Job burnout is a special type of work-related stress—a state of physical or emotional exhaustion that also involves a sense of reduced accomplishment and loss of personal identity. It has been related to adverse workplace conditions including unsafe, unhealthy, and stressful work environments. Some experts are critical of the term job burnout claiming it blames the victim. Rather they offer the term "moral injury" due to adverse working conditions.

Life expectancy Life expectancy is the average period that a person may be expected to live.

Member assistance programs (MAPs) MAPs are peer-based member assistance programs that were developed within the labor movement. MAPs emphasize the role of peer counselors—trained union members who volunteer their time to prevent drug abuse, motivate their coworkers who have drug abuse problems to accept referral for help, and support them when they return to work—union members helping each other to stay clean and sober.

Musculoskeletal disorders (MSDs) MSDs are soft tissue injuries caused by sudden or sustained exposure to repetitive motion, force, vibration, and awkward positions. These disorders can affect the muscles, nerves, tendons, joints, and cartilage in your upper and lower limbs, neck, and lower back.

National Institute for Occupational Safety and Health (NIOSH) NIOSH is the federal agency, located within the CDC, responsible for conducting research and making recommendations for the prevention of work-related injury and illness.

Occupation Occupation refers to the work a person does and consists of routine and nonroutine tasks necessary to perform their job.

Occupational health Occupational health refers to the identification and control of the risks arising from physical, chemical, biological, and ergonomic workplace hazards in order to prevent work-related disease.

Occupational illness An occupational illness results in disease due to exposure to chemical, biological, physical, or ergonomic health hazards. Ergonomic injuries that cause sprains and strains are considered occupational illnesses that are often associated with opioid use.

Occupational injury An occupational injury is bodily damage such as a cut, laceration, amputation, contusion, abrasion, or broken bones, damaged tissue, ligaments, or other body parts resulting from a sudden work-related traumatic incident.

Occupational safety and health Occupational safety and health is the discipline within public health that focuses on the identification and control of workplace hazards. The goal of occupational safety and health is to prevent workplace injury and illness and the related negative impacts on workers and employers.

Occupational Safety and Health Administration (OSHA) OSHA is the federal agency within the US Department of Labor with the responsibility of ensuring safety at work and a healthful work environment. OSHA's mission is to prevent work-related injuries, illnesses, and deaths. OSHA promulgates and enforces federal safety and health standards. Employers are required to comply with OSHA standards.

Occupational stress Occupational stress is psychological stress related to one's job. It may include ongoing or progressing stress an employee experiences due to the responsibilities, working conditions, work environment, organizational culture, or other pressures of the workplace.

Opioids Opioids are natural or synthetic chemicals that interact with opioid receptors on the nerve cells in the body and brain and reduce feelings of pain. They are a class of drugs that include prescription pain relievers, synthetic opioids, and heroin.

Opioid use disorder Opioid addiction is defined as a chronic, relapsing disorder characterized by compulsive drug seeking and use despite adverse consequences. It is considered a brain disorder, because it involves functional changes to brain circuits involved in reward, stress, and self-control, and those changes may last a long time after a person has stopped taking drugs.

Overdose Opioid overdose occurs when a person has physical and mental symptoms that occur after taking too many opioids causing excessive stimulation of the opiate pathway. This can lead to decreased respiratory function and possibly death.

Presenteeism Presenteeism is when a worker is present at work when they should not be, such as when they have an illness or family problem.

Public health model of prevention The public health model uses the principles of primary, secondary, and tertiary prevention. Primary prevention features interventions designed to prevent exposure from occurring. Secondary prevention occurs during the early stages of disease before onset of signs and symptoms. Tertiary prevention includes methods that aim to ameliorate the impact of disease once it has been established.

Recovery Recovery is defined as achieving sustained remission from the symptoms of substance use disorder.

Stigma Stigma is a mark of disgrace associated with a particular circumstance, quality, or person. Stigma related to drug use leads to treating users in a derogatory and discriminatory manner.

Substance use disorder Substance use disorders occur when the recurrent use of alcohol and/or drugs causes clinically significant impairment, including health problems, disability, and failure to meet major responsibilities at work, school, or home.

Substance use disorder treatment SUD treatment commonly consists of a combination of group and individual therapy sessions that focus on teaching those in recovery the skills needed to get and stay sober as well as how to navigate various situations without turning to drugs or alcohol. Additionally, medication treatments often play a significant role in in SUD treatment. Source: American Addiction Centers.

Tolerance Tolerance is the term used to explain that opioid users need to take increasingly higher dosages of drugs to achieve the same opioid effect.

Withdrawal Withdrawal relates to a user's growing tolerance. Most times, people who use opiates hit a level where they no longer feel pleasurable effects but continue to use because of the very painful physical and psychological symptoms that follow discontinuance of an addicting drug.

Zero tolerance policy These policies feature zero tolerance for drug use where anyone testing positive for drug use is terminated from employment. There may or may not be exceptions for prescription drug use where a licensed provider prescribes the medication.

Questions for Thought and Discussion

1. What are some of the major impacts of the opioid crisis on employers and the workplace?
2. What are some of the major impacts of the opioid crisis on workers and their families?
3. How does the public health model of prevention fit into a strategy for avoiding opioid misuse and addiction in the workplace?
4. Which industries and occupations are most affected by the opioid crisis and why?
5. What economic and public health disparities are associated with despair, chronic stress, and deaths from suicide, alcohol, and opioids?
6. What is ergonomics and why is prevention of musculoskeletal disorders a primary intervention in preventing opioid misuse?
7. What are examples of occupational stress factors that may increase risk of substance abuse?
8. What are the key criticisms of punitive workplace substance abuse policies?
9. What are the potential benefits of developing peer advocacy programs in the workplace?
10. What can be done to improve access to treatment and recovery programs in the workplace?

References

Bettinardi-Angres, K., Pickett, J., & Patrick, D. (2012). Substance use disorders and accessing alternative-to-discipline programs. *Journal of Nursing Regulation, 3*(2), 16–23. https://doi.org/10.1016/S2155-8256(15)30214-3.

Burris, S. (2018). Where next for opioids and the law? Despair, harm reduction, lawsuits, and regulatory reform. *Public Health Reports, 133*(1), 29–33. https://doi.org/10.1177/0033354917743500.

Cadiz, D. M., O'Neill, C., Schroeder, S., & Gelatt, V. (2015). Online education for nurse supervisors managing nurses enrolled in alternative-to-discipline programs. *Journal of Nursing Regulation, 6*(1), 25–32. https://doi.org/10.1016/S2155-8256(15)30006-5.

Caruso, C. C., Hitchcock, E. M., Dick, R. B., Russo, J. M., & Schmit, J. M. (2004). *Overtime and extended workshifts: Recent findings on injuries, illnesses, and health behaviors* (DHHS (NIOSH) Publication No. 2004-143). Retrieved from https://www.cdc.gov/niosh/docs/2004-143/pdfs/2004-143.pdf

Case, A., & Deaton, A. (2015). Rising morbidity and mortality in midlife among White non-Hispanic Americans in the 21st century. *PNAS, 112*(49), 15078–15083. https://doi.org/10.1073/pnas.1518393112. Retrieved from https://www.pnas.org/content/112/49/15078.

Centers for Disease Control and Prevention. (2019a). *Understanding the epidemic*. Retrieved August 8, 2019, from https://www.cdc.gov/drugoverdose/epidemic/index.html

Centers for Disease Control and Prevention. (2019b). *Picture of America: Prevention*. Retrieved August 8, 2019, from https://www.cdc.gov/pictureofamerica/pdfs/picture_of_america_prevention.pdf

Centers for Disease Control and Prevention. (2020a). *RX awareness*. Retrieved December 6, 2020, from https://www.cdc.gov/rxawareness/about/index.html

Centers for Disease Control and Prevention. (2020b). *Opioid overdose*. Retrieved December 6, 2020, https://www.cdc.gov/drugoverdose/opioids/prescribed.html

Center for the Organization for Economic Co-operation and Development (OECD). (2019). *Data, G-7 Annual hours of work 2017*. Retrieved from https://data.oecd.org/emp/hours-worked.htm

Connecticut Department of Public Health. (2018). *The opioid crisis and Connecticut's workforce: Updating your approach to employees suffering from addiction can preserve your greatest resource*. Retrieved from https://portal.ct.gov/-/media/Departments-and-Agencies/DPH/dph/environmental_health/occupationalhealth/Opioid-conference-writeup_FINAL-FINAL_11_28_18-(2).pdf?la=en

Council of Economic Advisers, Executive Office of the President. (2017). *Council of Economic Advisers report: The underestimated cost of the opioid crisis*. Retrieved from https://www.whitehouse.gov/sites/whitehouse.gov/files/images/The%20Underestimated%20Cost%20of%20the%20Opioid%20Crisis.pdf

Delaney, W., Grube, J. W., & Ames, G. M. (1998). Predicting likelihood of seeking help through the employee assistance program among salaried and union hourly employees. *Addiction, 93*(3), 399–410. https://doi.org/10.1046/j.1360-0443.1998.9333998.x.

Delp, L., Mojtahedi, Z., Sheikh, H., & Lemua, J. (2014). Legacy of struggle: The OSHA ergonomics standard and beyond, part II. *New Solutions, 24*(3), 365–389. https://doi.org/10.2190/NS.24.3.j.

Dembe, A. E., Erickson, J. B., Delbos, R. G., & Banks, S. M. (2005). The impact of overtime and long work hours on occupational injuries and illnesses: New evidence from the United States. *Occupational and Environmental Medicine, 62*(9), 588–597.

Dong, X. S., Fujimoto, A., Ringen, K., Stafford, E., Platner, J., Gittleman, J., & Wang, X. (2011). Injury underreporting among small establishments in the construction industry. *American Journal of Industrial Medicine, 54*(5), 339–349.

Economic Policy Institute. Lonnie Golden and Helene Jorgensen, (2002). *Time after time, mandatory overtime in the U.S. economy*. Retrieved August 8, 2019, from https://www.epi.org/

Enhancing OSHA's records audit process could improve the accuracy of worker injury and illness data. (2009). GAO-10-10. Retrieved October, 2020, from https://www.gao.gov/products/GAO-10-10

Fan, Z., Bonauto, D., Foley, M., & Silverstein, B. (2006). Underreporting of work-related injury or illness to workers' compensation: Individual and industry factors. *Journal of Occupational and Environmental Medicine, 48*(9), 914–922. https://doi.org/10.1097/01.jom.0000226253.54138.1e.

Franklin, G. M., Stover, B. D., Turner, J. A., Fulton-Kehoe, D., & Wickizer, T. M. (2008). Early opioid prescription and subsequent disability among workers with back injuries: The disability risk identification study cohort. *Spine, 33*, 199–204. https://doi.org/10.1097/BRS.0b013e318160455c.

Franklin, G., Sabel, J., Jones, C. M., Mai, J., Baumgartner, C , Banta-Green, C. J., et al. (2015). A comprehensive approach to address the prescription opioid epidemic in Washington State: Milestones and lessons learned. *American Journal of Public Health, 105*(3), 63–469. https://doi.org/10.2105/AJPH.2014.302367.

Golden, L., & Jorgens, H. (2002). *Time after time: Mandatory overtime in the U.S. economy* (Briefing paper#120). ECONOMIC Policy Institute. Retrieved from https://www.epi.org/publication/briefingpapers_bp120/

Gopireddy, M. M. R., Nisha, B., Prabhushankar, G., & Vishwambhar, V. (2016). Musculoskeletal morbidity among construction workers: A cross-sectional community-based study. *Indian Journal Occupational Environmental Medicine, 20*(3), 144–149. https://doi.org/10.4103/0019-5278.203134.

Hadland, S. E., Rivera-Aguirre, A., Marshall, B., & Cerdá, M. (2019). Association of pharmaceutical industry marketing of opioid products with mortality from opioid-related overdoses. *JAMA Network Open, 2*(1), e186007. https://doi.org/10.1001/jamanetworkopen.2018.6007.

Harduar Morano, L., Steege, A. L., & Luckhaupt, S. E. (2018). Occupational patterns in unintentional and undetermined drug-involved and opioid-involved overdose deaths-United States, 2007–2012. *Morbidity Mortality Weekly Report, 67*, 925–930. https://doi.org/10.15585/mmwr.mm6733a3.

Hemp, P. (2004). Presenteeism: At work—But out of it. *Harvard Business Review*. Retrieved from https://hbr.org/2004/10/presenteeism-at-work-but-out-of-it

Hersman, D. (2017). *How the prescription drug crisis is impacting American employers*. National Safety Council. Retrieved from https://www.nsc.org/Portals/0/Documents/NewsDocuments/2017/Media-Briefing-National-Employer-Drug-Survey-Results.pdf

Lassiter, M. (2015). Impossible criminals: The suburban imperatives of America's war on drugs, 2015. Published by Oxford University Press. https://doi.org/10.1093/jahist/jav243.

Lipscomb, J. A., Trinkoff, A. M., Geiger-Brown, J., & Brady, B. (2002). Work-schedule characteristics and reported musculoskeletal disorders of registered nurses. *Scandinavian Journal Work Environment Health, 28*(6), 394–401. https://doi.org/10.5271/sjweh.691.

Massachusetts Department of Public Health. (2018, August). *Opioid-related overdose deaths in Massachusetts by industry and occupation, 2011–2015*. Retrieved from https://www.mass.gov/files/documents/2018/08/15/opioid-industry-occupation.pdf

McLean, K. (2016). "There's nothing here": Deindustrialization as risk environment for overdose. *International Journal of Drug Policy, 29*, 19–26. https://doi.org/10.1016/j.drugpo.2016.01.009.

Monroe, T. B., Kenaga, H., Dietrich, M. S., Carter, M. A., & Cowan, R. L. (2013). The prevalence of employed nurses identified or enrolled in substance use monitoring programs. *Nursing Research, 62*(1), 10–15. https://doi.org/10.1097/NNR.0b013e31826ba3ca.

Moore, L. D., & Elkavich, A. (2008). Who's using and who's doing time? Incarceration, the war on drugs, and public health. *American Journal of Public Health, 98*(5), 782–786. https://doi.org/10.2105/AJPH.2007.126284. Retrieved from https://www.ncbi.nlm.nih.gov/pmc/articles/PMC2374804/pdf/0980782.pdf.

National Center for Health Statistics. (2017). *Health, United States, 2017: With special feature on mortality*. Hyattsville, 2018. Retrieved August 8, 2019, https://www.cdc.gov/nchs/hus/contents2017.htm#Table_014

National Institute for Occupational Safety and Health (NIOSH). (2019). *Hierarchy of Controls*. NIOSH. Retrieved August 8, 2019, from https://www.cdc.gov/niosh/topics/hierarchy/default.html

National Institute on Drug Abuse. (2019). *Drugs, brains, and behavior: The science of addiction*. National Institute on Drug Abuse. Retrieved from https://www.drugabuse.gov/publications/drugs-brains-behavior-science-addiction/drug-misuse-addiction

New York v. Purdue Pharma L.P., Purdue Pharma Inc, Purdue Frederick Co., Inc. (2018). Supreme Court of the State of New York, County of Suffolk. Retrieved from: https://ag.ny.gov/sites/default/files/400016_2018_the_people_of_the_stat_v_the_people_of_the_stat_summons_complaint_2.pdf

NIOSH. (2007, August). *Simple solutions ergonomics for construction workers* (DHHS (NIOSH) Publication No. 2007–122). Retrieved from https://www.cdc.gov/niosh/docs/2007-122/pdfs/2007-122.pdf?id=10.26616/NIOSHPUB2007122

O'Neill Hayes, T., & Manos, R. (2018). The opioid epidemic: Costs, causes, and efforts to fight it. *American Action Forum*. Retrieved from https://www.americanactionforum.org/research/opioidepidemic/

OSHA. (2013). *Safe patient handling programs, effectiveness and cost savings* (OSHA 3729–09/2013). Retrieved from https://www.osha.gov/Publications/OSHA3279.pdf

OSHA. *Ergonomics*. Retrieved December 6, 2020. https://www.osha.gov/SLTC/ergonomics/

Siddharthan, K., Nelson, A., Tiesman, H., & Chen, F. (2005). Cost effectiveness of a multifaceted program for safe patient handling. In K. Henriksen, J. B. Battles, E. S. Marks, (Eds.), *Advances in patient safety: From research to implementation issues, 3*. Retrieved from https://www.ahrq.gov/downloads/pub/advances/vol3/siddharthan.pdf

Statewide Peer Assistance for Nurses, "SPAN", New York State. (2017). Substance use among nurses and nursing students. *NYSNA, New York State Nurses Association, 14*(2). Retrieved from https://www.nysna.org/nursing-practice/statewide-peer-assistance-nurses#.WIEoM9-nFPY

Substance Abuse and Mental Health Services Administration. (2014). *Results from the 2013 National Survey on Drug Use and Health: Summary of National Findings* (NSDUH Series H-48, HHS Publication No. (SMA) 14-4863). Rockville: Substance Abuse and Mental Health Services Administration.

Substance Abuse and Mental Health Services Administration. (2016). *Results from the 2016 National Survey on Drug Use and Health: Summary of National Findings*. U.S. Department of Health and human Services.

Substance Abuse and Mental Health Services Administration. (2018). *Key substance use and mental health indicators in the United States: Results from the 2017 National survey on drug use and health* (HHS Publication No. SMA 18-5068, NSDUH Series H-53). Rockville: Center for Behavioral Health Statistics and Quality, Substance Abuse and Mental Health Services Administration. Retrieved October, 2020, from https://www.samhsa.gov/data/report/2017-nsduh-annual-national-report

Trust for America's Health. (2017). *Pain in the Nation: The drug, alcohol and suicide crises and the need for a national resilience strategy*. Retrieved October, 2020, from http://www.painin-thenation.org/assets/pdfs/TFAH-2017-PainNationRpt.pdf

U. S. Department of Health and Human Services. (2017). *Determination that a public health crisis exists*. Retrieved August 8, 2019, from https://www.hhs.gov/sites/default/files/opioid%20PHE%20Declaration-no-sig.pdf

U. S. Department of Health and Human Services. (2019). *What is the U.S. opioid epidemic?* Retrieved August 8, 2019, from https://www.hhs.gov/opioids/about-the-epidemic/index.html

US Bureau of Labor Statistics. (2018a). *Injuries, illnesses, and fatalities*. Retrieved August 8, 2019, from https://www.bls.gov/iif/

US Bureau of Labor Statistics. (2018b). *Employer-reported workplace injuries and illnesses*. Retrieved August 8, 2019, from https://www.bls.gov/news.release/archives/osh_11082018.pdf

Van Zee, A. (2009). The promotion and marketing of OxyContin: Commercial triumph, public health tragedy. *American Journal of Public Health, 99*(2), 221–227. https://doi.org/10.2105/AJPH.2007.131714.

Webster, B. S., Verma, S. K., & Gatchel, R. J. (2007). Relationship between early opioid prescribing for acute occupational low back pain and disability duration, medical costs, subsequent surgery and late opioid use. *Spine, 32*(19), 2127–2132. https://doi.org/10.1097/BRS.0b013e318145a731.

Weinmeyer, R. (2016). Safe patient handling laws and programs for health care workers. *American Medical Association Journal of Ethics, 18*(4), 416–421. https://doi.org/10.1001/journalofethics.2016.18.4.hlaw1-1604.

Weiss, R. M. (2010). Brinksmanship redux: Employee assistance programs' precursors and prospects. *Employee Responsibility and Rights Journal, 22*, 325–343. https://doi.org/10.1007/s10672-010-9144-0.

Working Partners Drug-Free Workforce Community Initiative. (2017). *Business survey*. Working Partners Systems, Inc. Retrieved from https://www.workingpartners.com/wp-content/uploads/2018/03/Preliminary-Highlights-Survey-Report.pdf

Zimmer, K. (2018). Follow the MAP: Helping craftworkers with substance abuse problems. *The Construction User*, 18–19. Retrieved from https://www.tauc.org/ihdp/tcu_spring_2018/EDE2F9809912E53AD5D01D0707F8396A/TCU_SPRING_2018.pdf

Chapter 3
Enhancing Cognitive Resilience in Adolescence and Young Adults: A Multidimensional Approach

Tara Rezapour, Shervin Assari, Namik Kirlic, Jasmin Vassileva, and Hamed Ekhtiari

1 Introduction

There has been a spiked interest in studying youth mental health problems, which affect nearly 20% of the total adolescent population globally (World Health Organization 2016). Many mental health disorders such as depression, suicide, eating disorders, and substance use disorders develop and manifest in adolescence and early adulthood (Chadda 2018; Jurewicz 2015; Nishida et al. 2016). Bohm and Clayton (2019) reported an increase in the number of adolescents aged 15–19 years who died of drug overdose from 831 in 2010 (3.8 per 100,000) to 873 in 2016 (4.1 per 100,000) in the United States. In 2018, the Substance Abuse and Mental Health Services Administration (SAMSHA) estimated 16.7% of adolescents (aged 12–17) were past-year illicit drug users, and about 1% were current heavy drinkers. Importantly, the prevalence of use increases significantly to 38.7% and 9.0% for illicit drug use and heavy alcohol, respectively in young adults (age 18–25 years). Risk-taking, using to enhance a positive state (positive reinforcement), using to

Hamed Ekhtiari, Tara Rezapour, Martin P. Paulus, and Robin L. Aupperle were involved with the ProCoRe program development.

T. Rezapour
Institute for Cognitive Science Studies, Tehran, Iran

S. Assari
University of Medicine and Science, Los Angeles, CA, USA

N. Kirlic · H. Ekhtiari (✉)
Laureate Institute for Brain Research, Tulsa, OK, USA
e-mail: hekhtiari@laureateinstitute.org

J. Vassileva
Department of Psychiatry, Institute for Drug and Alcohol Studies, Virginia Commonwealth University, Richmond, VA, USA

J. M. Croff, J. Beaman (eds.), *Family Resilience and Recovery from Opioids and Other Addictions*, Emerging Issues in Family and Individual Resilience,
https://doi.org/10.1007/978-3-030-56958-7_3

cope with a negative affect or stress (negative reinforcement), and lack of self-control against peer pressure are frequently reported as the individual-level motivations and causes for initial substance use (Donovan 2004; Dow and Kelly 2013; Titus et al. 2007). These reasons raise an urgent need and clarify that proper mental health programs can help protect adolescents from engagement in maladaptive behaviors in response to stressful, volatile, and risky situations.

1.1 Background

Neurobiological evidence supports a dual-system model to describe the inclination of adolescents toward risk-taking and emotion dysregulation (Hartley and Somerville 2015). According to this model, adolescence is a critical period associated with considerable developmental brain changes (Knudsen 2004; Spear 2000; Wetherill and Tapert 2013) characterized by continued structural and functional development of frontostriatal circuitry implicated in reward processing, impulse control, and emotion regulation (Bjork et al. 2007; Galvan et al. 2006, 2007). Frontostriatal circuitry is characterized by asynchronous pattern of development, with impulsive socioemotional striatal system maturing early and being disproportionately active relative to the later maturing top-down cognitive control system mediated by the prefrontal cortex (Blakemore and Robbins 2012; Casey et al. 2005; Clark and Winters 2002; Galvan et al. 2006; Giedd et al. 1999; Sowell et al. 2003). This asynchronous developmental pattern is related to increased risk-taking (Steinberg 2004), preference for immediate gratification over long-term gains (Claus et al. 2018; Stanger et al. 2013; Steinberg et al. 2009), discounting of future negative consequences (Steinberg et al. 2009), and exaggerated anticipation of positive outcomes of risky behaviors (Blakemore and Robbins 2012). These aberrant cognitive processes place adolescents and young adults at much higher risk for impulsive, risk-taking, or maladaptive coping behaviors including problematic substance use and development of substance use disorders (SUDs). The influence of genetic factors also increases across adolescence, as individuals have more freedom to express their genetic predispositions for risky behaviors such as alcohol use (Dick et al. 2016; McGue et al. 2006). Not surprisingly, adolescence is the peak age of onset for most psychiatric disorders (Lee et al. 2014).

The transition from childhood to adolescence is accompanied by alterations in different levels of individual, interpersonal and social goals and relationships (Jaworska and MacQueen 2015). Moving from a small-scale society (primary school) to the complicated adult world expose adolescents to a number of emotional challenges, evocative and risky situations (Casey et al. 2008). These stressful milestones, in turn, raise acute and chronic stress that may disturb physiological and psychological functions and increase the risk of development of serious pathological conditions (Dantzer et al. 2018; Franklin et al. 2012). Successful coping with these stressful conditions requires the ability to properly maintain mental homeostasis (e.g., emotion regulation and impulse control) as well as to actively employ effective problem-solving and decision-making strategies (Dray et al. 2014).

In this context, the concept of "resilience" in adolescence has received increased attention among developmental, cognitive, and clinical psychologists (Masten and Barnes 2018). Resilience includes various protective processes that enhance positive adaptation against stressful events (Liu et al. 2018). These factors and processes conceptualized as enabling assets and resources map on to individual, family, and culture (Masten and Barnes 2018). Therefore, resilience is defined as a dynamic capacity that buffers the impact of stress while keeping the balance in daily performance at both personal and societal levels (Wu et al. 2013). More recently, Masten and Barnes (2018) have extended this definition beyond individuals to include any complex adaptive system. According to their view, resilience could be applied to human organizations, ecosystems, economies, families, individuals as well as systems within an individual (e.g., immune system); however, in this chapter, we are focused on the resilience at the individual level.

Due to its multidimensional nature (Luthar et al. 2000; Wu et al. 2013), resilience can be discussed from different biological and psychological perspectives (Kahn et al. 2016; Liu et al. 2018). A common thread among studies of the neurophysiological and neuropsychological mechanisms for resilience is its trainable nature. Various training programs focusing on positive psychology (Victoria Cerezo et al. 2014), flexible interpretation (Loprinzi et al. 2011), stress reduction (Goodman and Schorling 2012; Mealer et al. 2014), self-management (McCraty andAtkinson 2012), self-awareness (Dyrbye et al. 2016), self-care techniques and self-regulation (Blair and Raver 2015), emotion regulation, and decision-making and social skills (Mache et al. 2016), have been proposed to improve resilience (Joyce et al. 2018). Specific training programs within these psychological frameworks show evidence of effectiveness in improving some aspects of resilience. Some examples are the Children's Resilience Program (Ambelu et al. 2019), Zippy's Friends (Clarke et al. 2014), You Can Do It! Education (Yamamoto et al. 2017), INSIGHTS (McClowry et al. 2010), and the Chicago School Readiness Project (CSRP)(Webster-Stratton et al. 2008).

In addition to the psychological approach to enhance resilience, a growing interest has emerged in the field of cognitive neuroscience toward studying resilience as a neurocognitive concept and defining its corresponding brain structures and functions (Richter et al. 2019). These studies have identified complex interactions between brain regions including the insula, cingulate cortex, hippocampus, nucleus accumbens, medial temporal lobe, and prefrontal cortex during emotion regulation and executive control (Iadipaolo et al. 2018; Liu et al. 2018; Russo et al. 2012; Wu et al. 2013). The balanced interaction between various neural regions, networks, and processes underlying "cognitive resilience" is a novel target for exploration. Neuroscience-based cognitive resilience is defined as a set of brain-derived abilities and processes for coping with the negative consequences of stress, adversity, and negative emotions while maintaining proper level of cognitive functions that are necessary for activities of daily living and avoiding high-risk behaviors (Ram et al. 2019). Cognitive resilience could be decomposed to various cognitive processes including working memory, response inhibition, cognitive flexibility, impulse control, reasoning, problem-solving, planning, and decision-making (Cambron et al.

2017; Nigg 2017). So, for the successful control of thoughts, emotions, impulses, and behaviors in the face of stressful events and evocative context, resilient adolescents should recruit a set of cognitive functions to encourage goal-attainment, positive adaptation, positive emotion, and adaptive decisions that will maximize long-term benefits (Artuch-Garde et al. 2017). From this perspective, a harmonized improvement in these cognitive processes will eventually result in more resilience.

However, only a few studies have indirectly targeted cognitive resilience through uni- and multimodal training of cognitive functions (e.g., attention, working memory, executive function) via curriculum-based interventions, exercise-based interventions, and social/interpersonal skills interventions among school-aged adolescents (Pandey et al. 2018). Far transfer effects of training (transfer the effects of training to nontrained tasks) (Rossignoli-Palomeque et al. 2018) include improvements in anxiety, teacher-reported behaviors, emotional symptoms (Roughan and Hadwin 2011), externalizing and internalizing behaviors (Riggs et al. 2006), impulsivity (Shure 1993), and physical aggression (Grossman et al. 1997).

In spite of the trainable components of cognitive resilience, we are not aware of any comprehensive cognitive resilience training programs for adolescents that target critical cognitive functions within a neuroscience-based framework and trigger experience-expectant plasticity (EEP) (Fuhrmann et al. 2015; Kerr et al. 2011). EEP is a type of neuroplasticity that refers to processes whereby the brain expects certain stimuli to learn new skills or competencies. Adolescence is typically known as a sensitive period, due to its high capacity for EEP (Fuhrmann et al. 2015). A program in which training modules are developed based on real-life conditions can trigger emotional or impulsive responses and train adaptive behaviors in a safe/controlled environment to develop EEP. In an ideal scenario, this program should provide adolescents with a neuroscience-based psychoeducation on cognitive components of resilience and instruct them on how to control their thoughts, emotions, and behaviors by implementing metacognitive and compensatory strategies within the context of real-life scenarios. Games and cartoons should make the educational materials engaging and entertaining for adolescents.

To fill this knowledge gap, in the following sections, we introduce a program that attempts to hierarchically train and integrate various dimensions of brain functions to build up cognitive resilience in adolescents. To our knowledge, this program is one of the first that takes a holistic approach to increase cognitive resilience of adolescents and young adults from a neurocognitive perspective.

1.2 Promoting Cognitive Resilience (ProCoRe) for Resilience

The "Promoting Cognitive Resilience" or ProCoRe is designed as a training program which targets cognitive functions involved in emotion regulation, impulse-control, learning-skills, stress-management, planning, flexibility, and problem-solving (Kent et al. 2015). ProCoRe is a paper-and-pencil program that integrates psychoeducational and game-based training. It includes 14 sessions. Each session takes around 90 min in a group setting. The curriculum content of each session is categorized into six interrelated sections including brain challenge scenario (narrative), brain concept (psychoeducation), brain exercise (game), brain box (metacognitive training), brain tip (compensatory strategies), and brain planner (time-management and activity monitoring). This categorization is consistent across all sessions and presented below:

1.2.1 Brain Challenge Scenarios

Each session starts with a cartoon-based scenario which narrates common problems that arise from deficits in the specific cognitive function targeted in the session (Debenham et al. 2020; Ekhtiari et al. 2017). These scenarios explain how these cognitive deficits impact our everyday life. The most important feature of this part of the curriculum is using simple and first-person narrative sentences to increase its self-reference effect. For example, in session 9, which focuses on "emotional memory," we use a comic cartoon (Fig. 3.1) and narrate this scenario:

> I also experience strong and detailed memories related to previous stressful events. Travelling through these negative memories can lead to negative emotions, such as guilt, anxiety, or hopelessness. I wish that I could erase those memories or ignore the emotions that come along with them.

1.2.2 Brain Concepts

This section explains the cognitive function discussed in the session in a psychoeducational context and describes how the deficits/disorders involving this cognitive function affect our real life (Labriole 2010). An example is emotional memory. It is

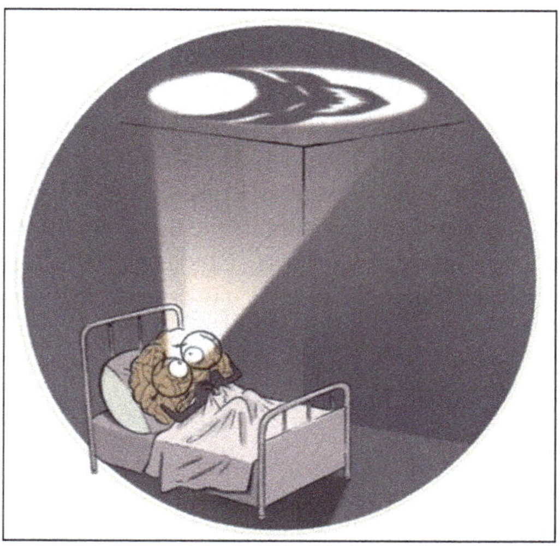

Fig. 3.1 Sample of a cartoon used in the brain challenge scenarios part (session related to emotional memory). (Cartoons by Naeem Tadayon, courtesy of Laureate Institute for brain research)

explained that emotionally salient information particularly with negative valence is more likely to be remembered for longer period of time rather than neutral information. Various interoceptive changes (e.g., heart rate) that may occur by recalling this information are also discussed. This section helps participants to gain awareness and insight about the underlying brain functions and the important roles they play in our day-to-day functioning.

1.2.3 Brain Tips

To efficiently manage cognitive resources, different evidence-based compensatory (i.e., stay focused strategies or mnemonics) or cognitive (i.e., eye gaze training or cognitive reappraisal) modulation strategies are provided as practical shortcuts that may help individuals to compensate for their limited cognitive and emotional resources especially in stressful conditions (Rossignoli-Palomeque et al. 2019; Vujovic and Urry 2018). For example, a strategy termed "expand your tunnel memory" is introduced to help participants expand their attentional span in face of distressing events and emotional memories. Using this brain tip may change the way that participants encode/recode information and reduce the intensity of the emotional response later when they recall the event or its memory. Such brain tips are usually followed by a relevant exercise (see next paragraph) (Breakout Box 3.1).

1.2.4 Brain Exercises

A set of game-based exercises is included in each session to engage relevant cognitive functions, as suggested by Kent et al. (2015). The additive architecture (see Fig. 3.2) is adapted to arrange the exercises across sessions, which means that each new session engages the previously activated cognitive functions plus the new one. The sessions have been ordered in such a way that they begin with the basic cognitive functions (e.g., attention and working memory) and gradually proceed to the higher-order functions (e.g., episodic future thinking and prospective memory). Figure 3.3 shows a sample of a brain exercise that practices tunnel memory technique in session 9 that added affective memory to the episodic memory introduced in session 8. This exercise is used to give participants an opportunity to experience how to reduce the vividness and emotionality of a central negative event in favor of the neutral details around. This exercise follows the preceding sections about the concept of tunnel memory and its modification strategies.

1.2.5 Brain Boxes

This section of the curriculum is a metacognitive training element which comes immediately after each brain exercise and informs participants about what cognitive functions were involved while they were doing the exercise/game (Matthews 2019;

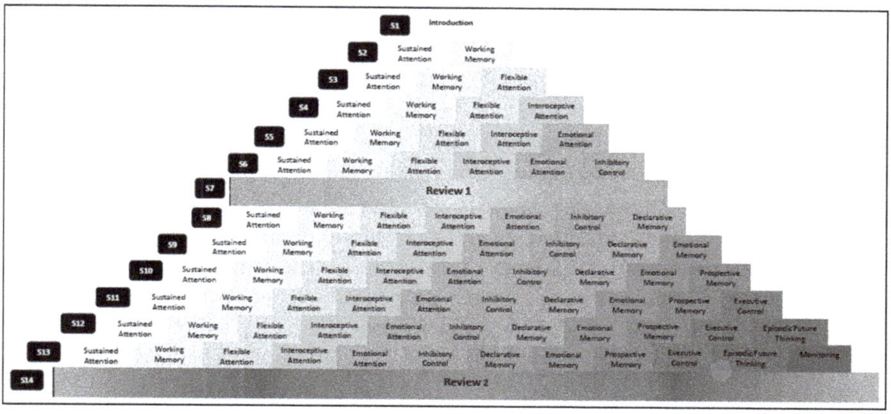

Fig. 3.2 Architecture of the ProCoRe for 14 sessions. In each session a new cognitive domain is added to the previous one in trainings and exercises (cumulative architecture). The brightness of color indicates the level of complexity of the cognitive modules. The basic modules (e.g., sustained attention) marked with bright colors and the complex ones marked with dark colors (e.g., monitoring)

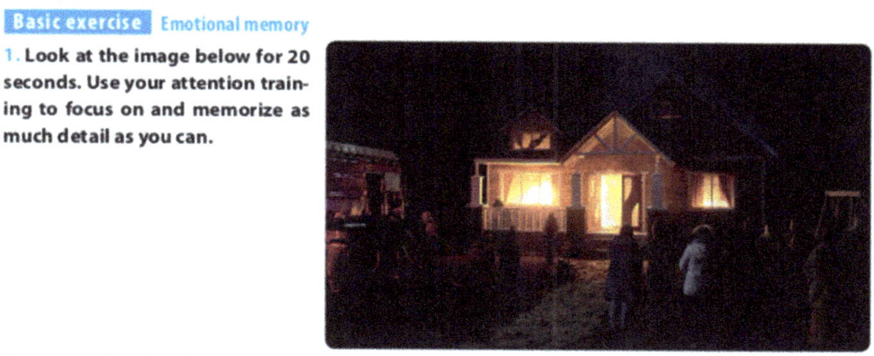
Basic exercise Emotional memory
1. Look at the image below for 20 seconds. Use your attention training to focus on and memorize as much detail as you can.

Fig. 3.3 Sample of emotional memory exercise used in the brain exercise part (session 9). In this exercise, participants should try to expand their attention to memorize the peripheral details of the main event, which is a house fire (e.g., the number of house windows), and recall them later

Pozuelos et al. 2019). Moreover, in this section, participants can find information about similar situations to the exercise that may happen in the context of real life. For example, the sample exercise mentioned above (Fig. 3.3) is similar to what happens in real life when we are faced with a stressful event (e.g., scene of a burning house in which someone gets hurt seriously) and how we can manipulate this type of memory to lessen the emotional intensity of the related visual memory.

1.2.6 Brain Planner

This section is a time-management, self-monitoring, or self-coaching part that trains participants how to monitor their emotions and behaviors as well as their progress toward their short-term and long-term goals, using a planner. This part of the curriculum is designed based on the work by (Plaete et al. 2016). In each session, participants are expected to do some specific activities related to the cognitive functions that are covered in each specific session. For example, in the session related to flexible attention, participants should record the experiences/events when they do more than one task at the same time or switch between different tasks in their real life. Participants should also write a short essay about their own experience of implementing the instructed compensatory strategies in their real life in the time between sessions.

In addition to the abovementioned features, participants are assigned with some homework. Homework for each session is expected to provide an opportunity for participants to further practice what they have learned (Foster et al. 2018).The brain planner mentioned above is considered part of the homework that should be completed before each session.

1.3 Cognitive Targets in ProCoRe Program

ProCoRe has been developed to train five major cognitive functions that play critical role in building cognitive resilience (i.e., attention, interoception, saliency processing, memory, and executive control) through stimulating goal-directed behaviors (Kent et al. 2015). These major cognitive functions and their subdivisions are hierarchically presented through 14 sessions (Fig. 3.2). The details of each cognitive module are described as below:

1.3.1 Attention

Various aspects of attention including focused and sustained attention, flexible attention, and emotional attention are targeted in ProCoRe. The "spotlight metaphor" is used to explain how the brain moves around and hunts for information in our environment and how this spotlight changes its size and direction in face of neutral and salient stimuli. During the training sessions, participants practice exercises that involve various aspects of attention and learn different brain tips including staying focused, mindfulness (Norris et al. 2018), paraphrasing, and self-talk (Hatzigeorgiadis and Galanis 2017). Therefore, the attention-related modules enable participants to stay focused and efficiently manage their attentional resources to capture important information and selectively filter irrelevant information.

1.3.2 Interoception

Following the sessions that are mainly focused on exteroceptive attention (sessions 2–3), the next modules target interoception and interoceptive attention. During session 4, participants are trained to use the spotlight (the metaphor used for attention) to focus on their internal signals (e.g., heart rate, muscle tension, gut feeling, and cold feeling in extremities) to consider these signals as a sign for specific emotion (e.g., anxious or anger) and use them to properly guide reciprocal behaviors (Khalsa et al. 2018). For example, they are trained to describe various physical and emotional changes that they may experience in face of an emotional event that may trigger impulsive decisions and/or actions (e.g., imagine that you see one of your close friends' pictures on Instagram hanging out at a party without telling you).

1.3.3 Saliency Processing

Several modules are devoted to explaining how saliency processing drives impulsive behaviors in face of incentive events and how this system becomes more prone to process stress-related stimuli more negatively (e.g., angry faces in crowd). The main goal pursued during these modules is to tune down the saliency attributed to emotional events by practicing strategies including gaze training (Sanchez-Lopez et al. 2019), behavioral activation (Dimidjian et al. 2006), and different types of reappraisal techniques (Cutuli 2014).

1.3.4 Memory

Different dimensions of memory processing are targeted next. These include declarative memory, emotional memory, and future (prospective) memory. In session 8, participants learn about episodic and semantic memories, their relationship to other cognitive domains introduced in previous sessions, and their importance in learning and daily life. Session 9 is devoted to emotional memory, which concerns specifically salient stressful information such as previous experiences of being rejected by friends. In this session, participants learn how to deal with these emotional memories and reduce their emotional responses to these memories through learning about memory reconsolidation (Beckers and Kindt 2017). Session 10 is focused on memory for future goals and plans or prospective memory. The aim of this session is to train participants how to create and imagine probable events that may happen in the future (Schacter et al. 2017). With developing prospective memories on how to handle risky or stressful scenarios, participants become better equipped to face potential challenges. This is a preparation for future sessions on self-control and decision-making where participants should recruit a goal-oriented mental imagery to anticipate the short- and long-term consequences of one's decision. During the memory-related sessions, various brain tips including mnemonic strategies, imagination, tunnel memory, and episodic future thinking are discussed. The overall aim of the memory-related sessions is to train participants for efficient use of memory for both past- and future-related memories, specifically those that may induce negative feelings once they are recalled or imagined.

1.3.5 Executive Control

In sessions 6, 10, 11, and 12, participants are trained in higher-order cognitive functions including inhibition, future thinking, planning, self-monitoring, problem-solving, and decision-making and learn how to recruit and integrate them with basic cognitive functions to face risky, emotional, and stressful scenarios. To depict the interaction between these functions, two acronyms as "WFI" (session 11) and "SLIDE" (sessions 12–13) are being introduced. The WFI acronym includes *W*orking memory, *F*lexibility, and *I*nhibition and aims to depict how participants can use these functions to control their impulsive and negative habitual behaviors. For example, participants are asked to use WFI terms to explain how they can control their impulsive choices and resist offers to use drugs or alcohol. These sessions consist of various brain tips, including development of "ready to go" plan and goal management training (Robertson 1996). The second acronym is "SLIDE" in which participants learn how to *S*pecify the problem, *L*ist possible solutions, *I*magine outcomes, *D*o the chosen solution, and *E*volve the solution (update future plans based on previous outcomes). To apply the SLIDE acronym, participants need to be trained in episodic future thinking, mental imagery, brainstorming, self-talk, and verbalization strategies. All these strategies improve forethought, planning, and anticipation skills. The most prominent feature of the sessions targeting self-control is using examples of real-life scenarios which are closely related to what they may really do in the context of their real life. For example, subjects are asked to imagine the following scenario and use SLIDE model to efficiently solve the problem: *"You have recently broken up with your very close friend. You have been feeling very down, lonely, and stressed since."*

1.4 EASICoRe Model in ProCoRe for Resilience

To depict how the five cognitive functions targeted in ProCoRe, i.e., attention, saliency processing, memory, interoception, and executive control, interact with each other in face of impulsive/emotional/stressful triggers, we have developed a heuristic model termed as "EASICoRe" in ProCoRe (Fig. 3.4). This neuroscience-informed model is used for both participants and trainers to frame their trainings through the ProCoRe program as an easily accessible heuristic.

According to this model, once participants are exposed to an impulsive, emotional, or stressful *E*nvironmental trigger, their *A*ttentional resources are allocated to process different aspects of the trigger (e.g., emotional and physical), while their memory is biased toward relevant emotional memories. By integrating the information from attention and memory, the evaluation system starts processing the *S*aliency

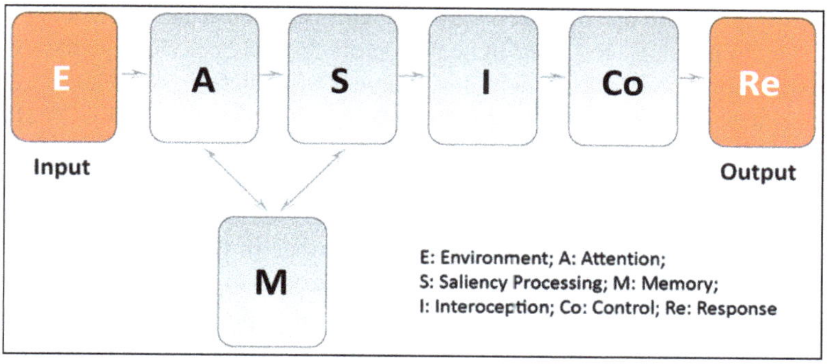

Fig. 3.4 EASICoRe model as a neuroscience informed conceptual framework indicates the interaction between cognitive modules in ProCoRe, which are activated in response to impulsive, emotional, and stressful triggers

of incoming information and comparing them with subjective goals/values based on available appraisal schemas. At this moment, various somatic signals originate from within the body transferring information related to bodily experiences (e.g., heart rate, respiration rate, pupillary dilation, flushing, perspiration, nociceptive reflexes). These *I*nteroceptive (somatic) signals contribute to emotional/appetitive experience and affect decision-making particularly under risk and uncertainty. Followed by evaluation, inhibitory *Co*ntrol may be activated to control impulsive desires and habits and direct behavior *Re*sponse toward more goal-oriented action. Therefore, EASICoRe can be considered as a neuroscience-informed framework which defines cognitive targets in the dynamic response to stressful, emotional, and appetitive cues. It is assumed that the proper functioning of each cognitive step as well as their interactions increases self-regulation and as a consequence improves resilience.

Due to the hierarchical structure of ProCoRe, in which cognitive modules are organized from the basic to the complex level, participants are presented with the EASICoRe model sequentially through the sessions and practice each module gradually in terms of real-life context. For example, by training with the attention-skills module, they learn how to use relevant brain tips to cope with attentional bias, or after learning the memory-related module, they start using relevant strategies to reduce negative feelings when they recall stressful events.

1.5 Public Health and Clinical Implication of ProCoRe for Drug Use Prevention

Enhancing resilience in order to increase adaptive behaviors in the face of stressful and emotional events can be extended to risky situations that may involve illicit drugs or alcohol use. To enhance the coverage for these situations, in an experiment, we added additional modules to ProCoRe to provide relevant pictorial and verbal scenarios. In the additional modules, participants learn through the EASICoRe model how substance use disorders develop with repeated drug use, which hijacks neural circuits normally involved in healthy motivational behaviors, such as eating, to motivate continued drug use and development of addiction. Additional cartoons and metaphors illustrate this change, such as the pictorial metaphor of "collapsed control room" used to indicate the effects of substance abuse on cognitive functions (Fig. 3.5). Moreover, to increase participants' knowledge about the effects of chronic substance use on the brain, additional modules provide neuroscience-informed educational materials that depict alterations in brain structure and function. The synergistic interaction of these additional substance use prevention modules to the ProCoRe and their effectiveness as a prevention intervention for substance use disorders need to be experimentally quantified by future studies.

1.6 Feasibility Study with ProCoRe

To examine the fit of ProCoRe in the real world, two lead authors in this chapter, Hamed Ekhtiari and Tara Rezapour with a group of collaborators, are running feasibility studies in two high schools as an educational curriculum on Iranian 11th graders during an academic year (2019–2020). ProCoRe consists of 14, 90-min group sessions which are manualized and mentored by trained coaches. The outcome measures are change of resilience and emotion regulation indexed by self-reports and neuropsychological assessments of executive functions (e.g., inhibition, working memory, and flexibility) from pre- to post intervention. Academic achievement measured by student's exam scores over the year and acceptability of the program are also assessed.

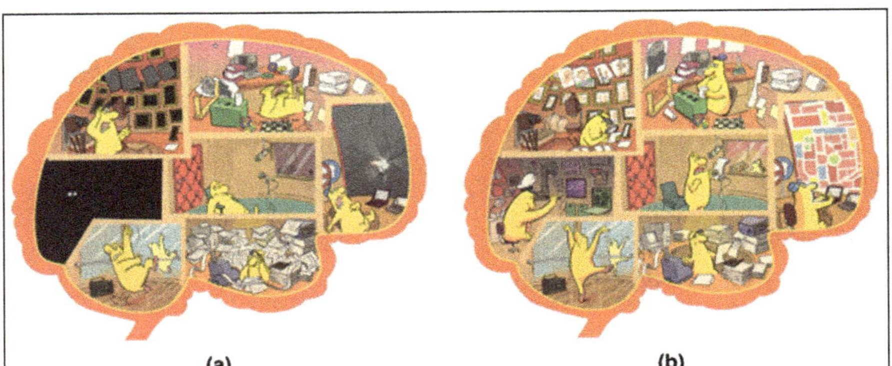

Fig. 3.5 Sample of a cartoon used in the neuroscience-informed education part related to drug addiction. Picture (**a**) indicated the changes in cognitive functions due to substance use and picture (**b**) indicates the cognitive functions in heathy brain

1.7 Challenges and Future Directions

From a neurocognitive perspective, cognitive resilience is embedded in a set of brain structures and cognitive functions which collectively contribute to the regulation of emotions, inhibition of impulses, motivation, and adaptive behaviors that result in positive outcomes (Fig. 3.6). In light of neuroplasticity and the trainable nature of cognitive functions (Ballesteros et al. 2018; Green and Bavelier 2008), ProCoRe has been developed as a modular training program inspired by a neuroscience-informed framework, EASICoRe. We hypothesize that this program improves cognitive resilience by targeting different cognitive functions involved in emotion regulation, impulse-control, learning, stress-management, flexibility, and problem-solving. Following the developmental phase of the program, the authors are testing the real-world efficacy of this training program with adolescents by focusing on measurable neurocognitive and behavioral markers. It would be critical to use a comprehensive neuropsychological battery, to test the efficacy of this program with diverse populations of youth at risk for substance misuse and other

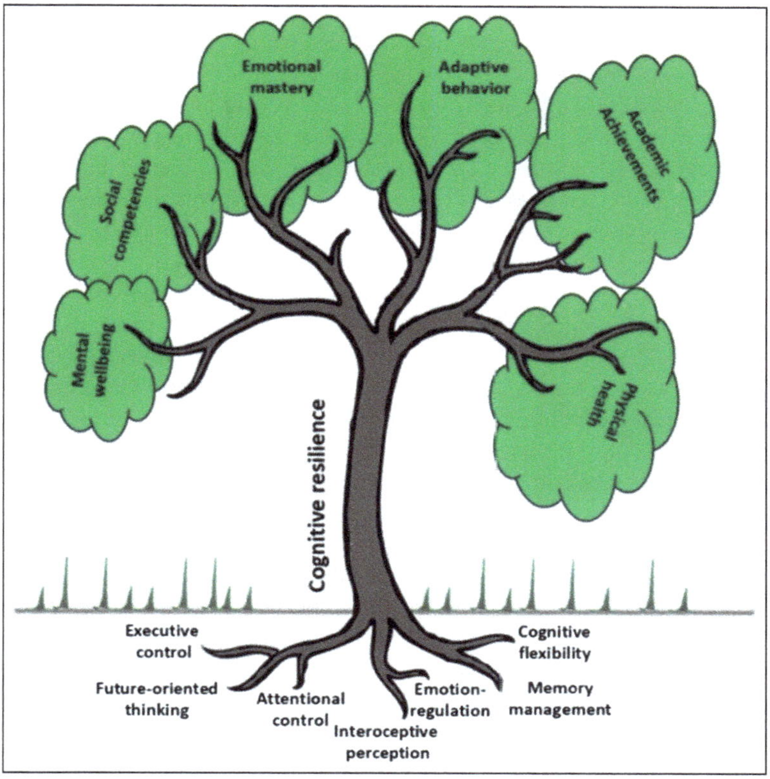

Fig. 3.6 Visualizing cognitive resilience with the concept of green tree (roots are metaphor for cognitive functions and branches are metaphor for outcomes)

maladaptive behaviors, including different racial and ethnic groups, those who were raised in poverty, individuals from single-parent families, as well as youth who identify as lesbian, gay, bisexual, and transgender (LGBT). Our next step is to prepare the computerized and cell-phone version of the ProCoRe to make it more accessible and interactive for individual applications. Translation of neuroscience evidence into practical applications makes ProCoRe trainings more real-life friendly and provides more opportunities for metacognitive awareness to reshape life skills. The ultimate goal is to scale the intervention to enhance population-level resilience of adolescents and young adults so they can avoid high-risk behaviors during times of stress. We welcome any collaborations to develop ProCoRe materials in different languages and assess the efficacy of the culturally adapted program in different communities.

Breakout Box 3.1. Focus on Practice

As a clinical psychologist, neuroscience provides me with a framework to better understand clients' experiences and behaviors. An understanding of neurodevelopment can be particularly helpful when working with adolescents in order to contextualize their behavior. It is also useful for communicating with parents the biological reasons for their child's moods and behaviors as well as what is normative and what is not. By relying on a solid neuroscientific basis as its foundation, Brain Gym can provide experiences that we know from research will help place teens on a path toward resilience and adaptive functioning. For example, the "brain tips" give adolescents tools they can use in their daily lives to strengthen important skills such as emotion regulation that in turn may contribute to positive development and maturation of cortical regions in the brain. Providing teens with psychoeducation on how our brains process information can help to both normalize their experiences as well as provide a means for them to gain more control over certain aspects of their experience, as seen through the example of emotion memory. Programs like Brain Gym may be helpful for teens dealing with substance use or other mental health problems because of how they integrate in-session and homework exercises with real-world examples. Youth are given the chance to practice the skills in a safe environment, often through doing paper-and-pencil activities that are quick and fun. These exercises can also make therapy more approachable. Activities such as these are nonthreatening for most youth and can help them interact with the material prior to trying to use the skills in a real-world situation where emotions and consequences are both much higher. Brain Gym is also highly structured, which is useful to keep adolescents focused and progressing through the program. The Brain Gym program is an effective example of how neuroscience findings can translate to practice in a way that is helpful to both providers and clients.

– Dr. Kara Kerr, Clinical Psychologist

Acknowledgements The authors would like to thank Seyed Naeim Tadayon Nabavi Fadafan (illustrator), Laleh Ziai (illustrator), and Mohsen Farhadi (graphic designer) for their contribution in creating cartoons and graphic design of ProCoRe program.

Glossary of Terms

Cognitive resilience A set of brain-derived abilities and processes for coping with the negative consequences of stress, adversity, and negative emotions while maintaining proper level of cognitive functions

Resilience A dynamic capacity that buffers the impact of stress while keeping the balance in daily performance at both personal and societal levels.

Transfer effect Transferring the effects of training to nontrained tasks.

Questions for Thought and Discussion

1. How does cognitive neuroscience approach explain the vulnerability of adolescents toward lack of control, risk-taking, and drug use behavior?
2. What does cognitive resilience mean to you? Write a one-two paragraph inspired by this chapter and explain why it is important to improve cognitive resilience.
3. What would be the outcome of improving cognitive resilience, particularly in adolescents? How would that change our current society?

References

Ambelu, A., Mulu, T., Seyoum, A., Ayalew, L., & Hildrew, S. (2019). Resilience dynamics after interventions made among school children of rural Ethiopia. *Heliyon, 5*(4), e01464. https://doi.org/10.1016/j.heliyon.2019.e01464.

Artuch-Garde, R., Gonzalez-Torres, M. D. C., de la Fuente, J , Vera, M. M., Fernandez-Cabezas, M., & Lopez-Garcia, M. (2017). Relationship between resilience and self-regulation: A study of Spanish youth at risk of social exclusion. *Frontiers in Psychology, 8*, 612. https://doi.org/10.3389/fpsyg.2017.00612.

Ballesteros, S., Voelcker-Rehage, C., & Bherer, L. (2018). Editorial: Cognitive and brain plasticity induced by physical exercise, cognitive training, video games, and combined interventions. *Frontiers in Human Neuroscience, 12*, 169. https://doi.org/10.3389/fnhum.2018.00169.

Beckers, T., & Kindt, M. (2017). Memory reconsolidation interference as an emerging treatment for emotional disorders: Strengths, limitations, challenges, and opportunities. *Annual Review of Clinical Psychology, 13*, 99–121. https://doi.org/10.1146/annurev-clinpsy-032816-045209.

Bjork, J. M., Smith, A. R., Danube, C. L., & Hommer, D. W. (2007). Developmental differences in posterior mesofrontal cortex recruitment by risky rewards. *The Journal of Neuroscience, 27*(18), 4839–4849. https://doi.org/10.1523/JNEUROSCI.5469-06.2007.

Blair, C., & Raver, C. C. (2015). School readiness and self-regulation: a developmental psychobiological approach. *Annual Review of Psychology, 66*, 711–731. https://doi.org/10.1146/annurev-psych-010814-015221.

Blakemore, S. J., & Robbins, T. W. (2012). Decision-making in the adolescent brain. *Nature Neuroscience, 15*(9), 1184–1191. https://doi.org/10.1038/nn.3177.

Bohm, M. K., & Clayton, H. (2019). Adolescent prescription opioid misuse, illicit opioid use and overdose. *Online Journal of Public Health Informatics, 11*(1), e422. https://doi.org/10.5210/ojphi.v11i1.9906.

Cambron, C., Kosterman, R., Catalano, R. F., Guttmannova, K., Herrenkohl, T. I., Hill, K. G., & Hawkins, J. D. (2017). The role of self-regulation in academic and behavioral paths to a high school diploma. *Journal of Developmental and Life-Course Criminology, 3*(3), 304–325. https://doi.org/10.1007/s40865-017-0066-5.

Casey, B. J., Galvan, A., & Hare, T. A. (2005). Changes in cerebral functional organization during cognitive development. *Current Opinion in Neurobiology, 15*(2), 239–244. https://doi.org/10.1016/j.conb.2005.03.012.

Casey, B., Jones, R. M., & Hare, T. A. (2008). The adolescent brain. *Annals of the New York Academy of Sciences, 1124*, 111–126.

Chadda, R. K. (2018). Youth & mental health: Challenges ahead. *The Indian Journal of Medical Research, 148*(4), 359–361. https://doi.org/10.4103/ijmr.IJMR_1585_18.

Clark, D. B., & Winters, K. C. (2002). Measuring risks and outcomes in substance use disorders prevention research. *Journal of Consulting and Clinical Psychology, 70*(6), 1207–1223. https://doi.org/10.1037/0022-006x.70.6.1207.

Clarke, A. M., Bunting, B., & Barry, M. M. (2014). Evaluating the implementation of a school-based emotional well-being programme: A cluster randomized controlled trial of Zippy's Friends for children in disadvantaged primary schools. *Health Education Research, 29*(5), 786–798. https://doi.org/10.1093/her/cyu047.

Claus, E. D., Feldstein Ewing, S. W., Magnan, R. E., Montanaro, E., Hutchison, K. E., & Bryan, A. D. (2018). Neural mechanisms of risky decision making in adolescents reporting frequent alcohol and/or marijuana use. *Brain Imaging and Behavior, 12*(2), 564–576. https://doi.org/10.1007/s11682-017-9723-x.

Cutuli, D. (2014). Cognitive reappraisal and expressive suppression strategies role in the emotion regulation: An overview on their modulatory effects and neural correlates. *Frontiers in Systems Neuroscience, 8*, 175. https://doi.org/10.3389/fnsys.2014.00175.

Dantzer, R., Cohen, S., Russo, S. J., & Dinan, T. G. (2018). Resilience and immunity. *Brain, Behavior, and Immunity, 74*, 28–42. https://doi.org/10.1016/j.bbi.2018.08.010.

Debenham, J., Birrell, L., Champion, K., Askovic, M., & Newton, N. (2020). A pilot study of a neuroscience-based, harm minimisation programme in schools and youth centres in Australia. *BMJ Open, 10*(2), e033337. https://doi.org/10.1136/bmjopen-2019-033337.

Dick, D. M., Adkins, A. E., & Kuo, S. I. (2016). Genetic influences on adolescent behavior. *Neuroscience and Biobehavioral Reviews, 70*, 198–205. https://doi.org/10.1016/j.neubiorev.2016.07.007.

Dimidjian, S., Hollon, S. D., Dobson, K. S., Schmaling, K. B., Kohlenberg, R. J., Addis, M. E., et al. (2006). Randomized trial of behavioral activation, cognitive therapy, and antidepressant medication in the acute treatment of adults with major depression. *Journal of Consulting and Clinical Psychology, 74*(4), 658–670. https://doi.org/10.1037/0022-006X.74.4.658.

Donovan, J. E. (2004). Adolescent alcohol initiation: A review of psychosocial risk factors. *Journal of Adolescent Health, 35*(6), 529. e527–529. e518.

Dow, S. J., & Kelly, J. F. (2013). Listening to youth: Adolescents' reasons for substance use as a unique predictor of treatment response and outcome. *Psychology of Addictive Behaviors, 27*(4), 1122.

Dray, J., Bowman, J., Freund, M., Campbell, E., Wolfenden, L., Hodder, R. K., & Wiggers, J. (2014). Improving adolescent mental health and resilience through a resilience-based intervention in schools: Study protocol for a randomised controlled trial. *Trials, 15*(289), 1–9.

Dyrbye, L. N., West, C. P., Richards, M. L., Ross, H. J., Satele, D., & Shanafelt, T. D. (2016). A randomized, controlled study of an online intervention to promote job satisfaction and well-being among physicians. *Burnout Research, 3*(3), 69–75. https://doi.org/10.1016/j.burn.2016.06.002.

Ekhtiari, H., Rezapour, T., Aupperle, R. L., & Paulus, M. P. (2017). Neuroscience-informed psychoeducation for addiction medicine: A neurocognitive perspective. *Progress in Brain Research, 235*, 239–264. https://doi.org/10.1016/bs.pbr.2017.08.013.

Foster, E. R., Spence, D., & Toglia, J. (2018). Feasibility of a cognitive strategy training intervention for people with Parkinson's disease. *Disability and Rehabilitation, 40*(10), 1127–1134. https://doi.org/10.1080/09638288.2017.1288275.

Franklin, T. B., Saab, B. J., & Mansuy, I. M. (2012). Neural mechanisms of stress resilience and vulnerability. *Neuron, 75*(5), 747–761. https://doi.org/10.1016/j.neuron.2012.08.016.

Fuhrmann, D., Knoll, L. J., & Blakemore, S. -J. (2015). Adolescence as a sensitive period of brain development. *Trends in Cognitive Sciences, 19*, 558–566. https://doi.org/10.1016/j.tics.2015.07.008

Galvan, A., Hare, T. A., Parra, C. E., Penn, J., Voss, H., Glover, G., & Casey, B. J. (2006). Earlier development of the accumbens relative to orbitofrontal cortex might underlie risk-taking behavior in adolescents. *The Journal of Neuroscience, 26*(25), 6885–6892. https://doi.org/10.1523/JNEUROSCI.1062-06.2006.

Galvan, A., Hare, T., Voss, H., Glover, G., & Casey, B. J. (2007). Risk-taking and the adolescent brain: Who is at risk? *Developmental Science, 10*(2), F8–F14. https://doi.org/10.1111/j.1467-7687.2006.00579.x.

Giedd, J., Blumenthal, J., Jeffries, N. O., Castellanos, F. X., Liu, H., Zijdenbos, A., Paus, T., Evans, A. C., & Rapoport, J. L. (1999). Brain development during childhood and adolescence: a longitudinal MRI study. *Nature Neuroscience, 2*(10), 861–863.

Goodman, M. J., & Schorling, J. B. (2012). A mindfulness course decreases burnout and improves well-being among healthcare providers. *International Journal of Psychiatry in Medicine, 43*(2), 119–128. https://doi.org/10.2190/PM.43.2.b.

Green, C. S., & Bavelier, D. (2008). Exercising your brain: A review of human brain plasticity and training-induced learning. *Psychology and Aging, 23*(4), 692–701. https://doi.org/10.1037/a0014345.

Grossman, D., Neckerman, H. J., Koepsell, T. D., Liu, P. Y., Asher, K. N., Beland, K., Frey, K., & Rivara, F. P. (1997). Effectiveness of a violence prevention curriculum among children in elementary school. A randomized controlled trial. *JAMA. 277*(20), 1605–1611.

Hartley, C. A., & Somerville, L. H. (2015). The neuroscience of adolescent decision-making. *Current Opinion in Behavioral Sciences, 5*, 108–115. https://doi.org/10.1016/j.cobeha.2015.09.004.

Hatzigeorgiadis, A., & Galanis, E. (2017). Self-talk effectiveness and attention. *Current Opinion in Psychology, 16*, 138–142. https://doi.org/10.1016/j.copsyc.2017.05.014.

Iadipaolo, A. S., Marusak, H. A., Paulisin, S. M., Sala-Hamrick, K., Crespo, L. M., Elrahal, F., et al. (2018). Distinct neural correlates of trait resilience within core neurocognitive networks in at-risk children and adolescents. *Neuroimage Clinical, 20*, 24–34. https://doi.org/10.1016/j.nicl.2018.06.026.

Jaworska, N., & MacQueen, G. (2015). Adolescence as a unique developmental period. *Journal of Psychiatry & Neuroscience, 40*(5), 291–293. https://doi.org/10.1503/jpn.150268.

Joyce, S., Shand, F., Tighe, J., Laurent, S. J., Bryant, R. A., & Harvey, S. B. (2018). Road to resilience: a systematic review and meta-analysis of resilience training programmes and interventions. *BMJ Open, 8*(6), e017858. https://doi.org/10.1136/bmjopen-2017-017858.

Jurewicz, I. (2015). Mental health in young adults and adolescents—Supporting general physicians to provide holistic care. *Clinical Medicine (London, England), 15*(2), 151–154.

Kahn, J. R., Collinge, W., & Soltysik, R. (2016). Post-9/11 veterans and their partners improve mental health outcomes with a self-directed mobile and web-based wellness training program: A randomized controlled trial. *Journal of Medical Internet Research, 18*(9), e255. https://doi.org/10.2196/jmir.5800.

Kent, M., Rivers, C. T., & Wrenn, G. (2015). Goal-Directed Resilience in Training (GRIT): A biopsychosocial model of self-regulation, executive functions, and personal growth (Eudaimonia) in evocative contexts of PTSD, obesity, and chronic pain. *Behav Sci (Basel), 5*(2), 264–304. https://doi.org/10.3390/bs5020264.

Kerr, A. L., Cheng, S. Y., & Jones, T. A. (2011). Experience-dependent neural plasticity in the adult damaged brain. *Journal of communication disorders, 44*(5), 538–548. https://doi.org/10.1016/j.jcomdis.2011.04.011

Khalsa, S. S., Adolphs, R., Cameron, O. G., Critchley, H. D., Davenport, P. W., Feinstein, J. S., et al. (2018). Interoception and mental health: A roadmap. *Biol Psychiatry Cogn Neurosci Neuroimaging, 3*(6), 501–513. https://doi.org/10.1016/j.bpsc.2017.12.004.

Knudsen, E. (2004). Sensitive periods in the development of the brain and behavior. *Journal of Cognitive Neuroscience, 16*(8), 1412–1425.

Labriole, M. (2010). Promoting brain-science literacy in the K-12 classroom by Michaela Labriole. *Cerebrum: The Dana Forum on Brain Science, 15*, 1–14.

Lee, F. S., Heimer, H., Giedd, J. N., Lein, E. S., Sestan, N., Weinberger, D. R., & Casey, B. J. (2014). Mental health. Adolescent mental health—opportunity and obligation. *Science, 346*(6209), 547–549. https://doi.org/10.1126/science.1260497.

Liu, H., Zhang, C., Ji, Y., & Yang, L. (2018). Biological and psychological perspectives of resilience: Is it possible to improve stress resistance? *Frontiers in Human Neuroscience, 12*, 326. https://doi.org/10.3389/fnhum.2018.00326.

Loprinzi, C. E., Prasad, K., Schroeder, D. R., & Sood, A. (2011). Stress Management and Resilience Training (SMART) program to decrease stress and enhance resilience among breast cancer survivors: A pilot randomized clinical trial. *Clinical Breast Cancer, 11*(6), 364–368.

Luthar, S. S., Cicchetti, D., & Becker, B. (2000). The construct of resilience: A critical evaluation and guidelines for future work. *Child Development, 71*(3), 543–562.

Mache, S., Bernburg, M., Baresi, L., & Groneberg, D. A. (2016). Evaluation of self-care skills training and solution-focused counselling for health professionals in psychiatric medicine: A pilot study. *International Journal of Psychiatry in Clinical Practice, 20*(4), 239–244. https://doi.org/10.1080/13651501.2016.1207085.

Masten, A. S., & Barnes, A. J. (2018). Resilience in children: Developmental perspectives. *Children (Basel), 5*(7). https://doi.org/10.3390/children5070098.

Matthews, G., Panganiban, A. R., Wells, A., Wohleber, R. W., & Reinerman-Jones, L. E. (2019). Metacognition, hardiness, and grit as resilience factors in Unmanned Aerial Systems (UAS) operations: A simulation study. *Frontiers in Psychology, 10*, 640. https://doi.org/10.3389/fpsyg.2019.00640.

McClowry, S. G., Snow, D. L., Tamis-Lemonda, C. S., & Rodriguez, E. T. (2010). Testing the efficacy of INSIGHTS on student disruptive behavior, classroom management, and student competence in inner city primary grades. *School Mental Health, 2*(1), 23–35. https://doi.org/10.1007/s12310-009-9023-8.

McCraty, R., & Atkinson, M. (2012). Resilience training program reduces physiological and psychological stress in police officers. *Glob Adv Health Med, 1*(5), 44–66.

McGue, M., Iacono, W., & Krueger, R. (2006). The association of early adolescent problem behavior and adult psychopathology: A multivariate behavioral genetic perspective. *Behavior Genetics, 36*(4), 591–602.

Mealer, M., Conrad, D., Evans, J., Jooste, K., Solyntjes, J., Rothbaum, B., & Moss, M. (2014). Feasibility and acceptability of a resilience training program for intensive care unit nurses. *American Journal of Critical Care, 23*(6), e97–e105. https://doi.org/10.4037/ajcc2014747.

Nigg, J. T. (2017). Annual research review: On the relations among self-regulation, self-control, executive functioning, effortful control, cognitive control, impulsivity, risk-taking, and inhibition for developmental psychopathology. *Journal of Child Psychology and Psychiatry, 58*(4), 361–383. https://doi.org/10.1111/jcpp.12675.

Nishida, A., Richards, M., & Stafford, M. (2016). Prospective associations between adolescent mental health problems and positive mental wellbeing in early old age. *Child and Adolescent Psychiatry and Mental Health, 10*, 12. https://doi.org/10.1186/s13034-016-0099-2.

Norris, C. J., Creem, D., Hendler, R., & Kober, H. (2018). Brief mindfulness meditation improves attention in novices: evidence from ERPs and moderation by neuroticism. *Frontiers in Human Neuroscience, 12*, 315. https://doi.org/10.3389/fnhum.2018.00315.

Pandey, A., Hale, D., Das, S., Goddings, A. L., Blakemore, S. J., & Viner, R. M. (2018). Effectiveness of universal self-regulation-based interventions in children and adolescents: A systematic review and meta-analysis. *JAMA Pediatrics, 172*(6), 566–575.

Plaete, J., De Bourdeaudhuij, I., Verloigne, M., & Crombez, G. (2016). The use and evaluation of self-regulation techniques can predict health goal attainment in adults: an explorative study. *PeerJ, 4*, e1666. https://doi.org/10.7717/peerj.1666.

Pozuelos, J. P., Combita, L. M., Abundis, A., Paz-Alonso, P. M., Conejero, A., Guerra, S., & Rueda, M. R. (2019). Metacognitive scaffolding boosts cognitive and neural benefits following executive attention training in children. *Developmental Science, 22*(2), e12756. https://doi.org/10.1111/desc.12756.

Ram, D., Chandran, S., Sadar, A., & Gowdappa, B. (2019). Correlation of cognitive resilience, cognitive flexibility and impulsivity in attempted suicide. *Indian Journal of Psychological Medicine, 41*(4), 362–367. https://doi.org/10.4103/IJPSYM.IJPSYM_189_18.

Richter, A., Kramer, B., Diekhof, E. K., & Gruber, O. (2019). Resilience to adversity is associated with increased activity and connectivity in the VTA and hippocampus. *Neuroimage Clinical, 23*, 101920. https://doi.org/10.1016/j.nicl.2019.101920.

Riggs, N., Greenberg, M. T., Kusché, C. A., & Pentz, M. A. (2006). The mediational role of neurocognition in the behavioral outcomes of a social-emotional prevention program in elementary school students: Effects of the PATHS Curriculum. *Prevention Science, 7*(1), 91–102.

Robertson, I. H. (1996). Goal management training: a clinical manual. Cambridge: PsyConsult; [Google Scholar].

Rossignoli-Palomeque, T., Perez-Hernandez, E., & Gonzalez-Marques, J. (2018). Brain training in children and adolescents: Is it scientifically valid? *Frontiers in Psychology, 9*, 565. https://doi.org/10.3389/fpsyg.2018.00565.

Rossignoli-Palomeque, T., Quiros-Godoy, M., Perez-Hernandez, E., & Gonzalez-Marques, J. (2019). Schoolchildren's compensatory strategies and skills in relation to attention and executive function app training. *Frontiers in Psychology, 10*, 2332. https://doi.org/10.3389/fpsyg.2019.02332.

Roughan, L., & Hadwin, J. A. (2011). The impact of working memory training in young people with social, emotional and behavioural difficulties. *Learning and Individual Differences, 21*(6), 759–764. https://doi.org/10.1016/j.lindif.2011.07.011.

Russo, S. J., Murrough, J. W., Han, M. H., Charney, D. S., & Nestler, E. J. (2012). Neurobiology of resilience. *Nature Neuroscience, 15*(11), 1475–1484. https://doi.org/10.1038/nn.3234.

Sanchez-Lopez, A., Everaert, J., Van Put, J., De Raedt, R., & Koster, E. H. W. (2019). Eye-gaze contingent attention training (ECAT): Examining the causal role of attention regulation in reappraisal and rumination. *Biological Psychology, 142*, 116–125. https://doi.org/10.1016/j.biopsycho.2019.01.017.

Schacter, D. L., Benoit, R. G., & Szpunar, K. K. (2017). Episodic future thinking: Mechanisms and functions. *Current Opinion in Behavioral Sciences, 17*, 41–50. https://doi.org/10.1016/j.cobeha.2017.06.002.

Shure, M. B. (1993). I Can Problem Solve (ICPS): Interpersonal cognitive problem solving for young children. *Early Child Development and Care, 96*(1), 49–64. https://doi.org/10.1080/0300443930960106.

Sowell, E. R., Peterson, B. S., Thompson, P. M., Welcome, S. E., Henkenius, A. L., & Toga, A. W. (2003). Mapping cortical change across the human life span. *Nature Neuroscience, 6*(3), 309–315. https://doi.org/10.1038/nn1008.

Spear, L. (2000). The adolescent brain and age-related behavioral manifestations. *Neuroscience and Biobehavioral Reviews, 24*(4), 417–463.

Stanger, C., Budney, A. J., & Bickel, W. K. (2013). A developmental perspective on neuroeconomic mechanisms of contingency management. *Psychology of Addictive Behaviors, 27*(2), 403–415. https://doi.org/10.1037/a0028748.

Steinberg, L. (2004). Risk taking in adolescence: What changes, and why? *Annals of the New York Academy of Sciences, 1021*, 51–58.

Steinberg, L., Graham, S., O'Brien, L., Woolard, J., Cauffman, E., & Banich, M. (2009). Age differences in future orientation and delay discounting. *Child Development, 80*(1), 28–44.

Titus, J. C., Godley, S. H., & White, M. K. (2007). A post-treatment examination of adolescents' reasons for starting, quitting, and continuing the use of drugs and alcohol. *Journal of Child & Adolescent Substance Abuse, 16*(2), 31–49.

Victoria Cerezo, M., Ortiz-Tallo, M., Cardenal, V., & De La Torre-Luque, A. (2014). Positive psychology group intervention for breast cancer patients: A randomised trial. *Psychological Reports, 115*(1), 44–64. https://doi.org/10.2466/15.20.PR0.115c17z7.

Vujovic, L., & Urry, H. L. (2018). Emotion Regulation compensation following situation selection failure. *Scientific Reports, 8*(1), 5411. https://doi.org/10.1038/s41598-018-23654-2.

Webster-Stratton, C., Jamila Reid, M., & Stoolmiller, M. (2008). Preventing conduct problems and improving school readiness: Evaluation of the Incredible Years Teacher and Child Training Programs in high-risk schools. *Journal of Child Psychology and Psychiatry, 49*(5), 471–488. https://doi.org/10.1111/j.1469-7610.2007.01861.x.

Wetherill, R., & Tapert, S. F. (2013). Adolescent brain development, substance use, and psychotherapeutic change. *Psychology of Addictive Behaviors, 27*(2), 393–402. https://doi.org/10.1037/a0029111.

WHO (2016). WHO| Child and Adolescent Mental Health. WHO. World Health Organization. Available online at: http://www.who.int/mental_health/maternalchild/child_adolescent/en/.

Wu, G., Feder, A., Cohen, H., Kim, J. J., Calderon, S., Charney, D. S., & Mathe, A. A. (2013). Understanding resilience. *Frontiers in Behavioral Neuroscience, 7*, 10. https://doi.org/10.3389/fnbeh.2013.00010.

Yamamoto, T., Matsumoto, Y., & Bernard, M. E. (2017). Effects of the cognitive-behavioral You Can Do It! Education program on the resilience of Japanese elementary school students: A preliminary investigation. *International Journal of Educational Research, 86*, 50–58. https://doi.org/10.1016/j.ijer.2017.08.006.

Chapter 4
Family-Centered Care Approaches for Neonatal Abstinence Syndrome: Caring for Mothers and Infants

Lucia Ciciolla, Gina Erato, Samantha Addante, Mira Armans, and Ashley Quigley

1 Literature Review

1.1 Clinical Presentation and Features of NAS

NAS is a complex syndrome characterized by signs and symptoms of substance withdrawal, with primary involvement of the central and autonomic nervous systems and the gastrointestinal system (Jansson and Velez 2012). Signs and symptoms of NAS can vary widely in severity and the systems affected, but are generally characterized as neurobehavioral dysregulation, and may include tremors, increased muscle tone, excessive and/or high-pitched cry, excessive motor movements, seizures, diarrhea, vomiting, difficulty feeding, excessive sucking, hyperphagia, hyper-irritability, temperature instability and fever, sweating, sneezing, yawning, and increased respiratory rate. Infants with NAS may have difficulty gaining weight and trouble sleeping, and are notoriously difficult to soothe. Signs of the syndrome often begin in the first few days after birth, with some infants experiencing only a short but intense initial phase lasting for 1 to 2 weeks, and others having this initial phase followed by a chronic and relapsing course lasting several weeks to a few months (Kocherlakota 2014). Importantly, NAS is rarely a cause of infant death, and most infants are discharged from the hospital in healthy condition (Abdel-Latif et al. 2007).

The term "mother" is used throughout this chapter both specifically and generically – specifically, because the majority of the literature on substance-exposed infants and NAS has focused on mothers and, generically, to stand more broadly for parents and primary caregivers of infants. It should be noted however, that not all birthing persons identify as mothers or women.

L. Ciciolla (✉) · G. Erato · S. Addante · M. Armans · A. Quigley
Department of Psychology, Oklahoma State University, Stillwater, OK, USA
e-mail: lucia.ciciolla@okstate.edu

J. M. Croff, J. Beaman (eds.), *Family Resilience and Recovery from Opioids and Other Addictions*, Emerging Issues in Family and Individual Resilience,
https://doi.org/10.1007/978-3-030-56958-7_4

NAS occurs as a result of the sudden discontinuation of fetal exposure to substances that were used or abused by the mother during pregnancy (Kocherlakota 2014). Although opioids are the most common substance associated with NAS, including heroin, methadone, buprenorphine, and prescription opioid medications, fetal exposure to other substance have also been implicated, including nicotine, benzodiazepines, methamphetamines, and antidepressant medications, including selective serotonin reuptake inhibitors (SSRIs) and tricyclic antidepressants (TCAs).

Exposure to more than one type of substance can also alter the onset of NAS and potentiate the severity of the symptoms. Differences in the onset, severity, and course of NAS are not well understood but may vary based on the type and combination of substances used, pharmacological properties, placental transferability, dosage, duration and timing of exposure, and the total accumulation of exposure during pregnancy (Kocherlakota 2014; Patrick et al. 2016). Known risk factors associated with increased severity and/or intensity of NAS include infants born at term, good birth weight, maternal polysubstance use (in particular, benzodiazepines, and possibly SSRIs, in combination with other substances), maternal methadone use, maternal smoking, infant genetic predisposition for delayed drug metabolism, and male gender (Kocherlakota 2014).

1.2 *Epidemiology*

According to data from the Healthcare Cost and Utilization Project (HCUP), the overall incidence rate of NAS was 6.7 per 1000 in-hospital births in 2016, totaling approximately one baby being diagnosed with NAS every 19 min in the United States, or nearly 80 newborns diagnosed every day and 30,000 diagnosed each year (Centers for Disease Control and Prevention 2020; Strahan et al. 2020). The increase in the incidence of NAS over the past several decades is associated with the increased prevalence of substance use during pregnancy, particularly opioid use (McQueen and Murphy-Oikonen 2016). Based on data from the National Surveys on Drug Use and Health (NSDUHs) from 2016 to 2017, approximately 1.4% of pregnant women were reported to misuse opioids in the prior month, including pain relievers and heroin (Center for Behavioral Health Statistics and Quality 2018), and the percentage of pregnant women entering treatment who reported any prescription opioid misuse increased from 2% to 28% between 1992 and 2010 (Martin et al. 2015). Between 1999 and 2014, the prevalence of opioid use disorder among pregnant women in the United States increased more than threefold (Haight et al. 2018), and the incidence of NAS diagnoses increased more than fivefold across a 10-year period (2004–2014) (Winkelman et al. 2018).

It should be noted that although the incidence of opioid misuse and NAS has increased across all communities, mothers and infants from low-income communities and those covered by public insurance have been disproportionately affected (Winkelman et al. 2018). Increasing incidence of NAS has followed geographic trends associated with the US opioid crisis, with the highest rates of NAS reported in states with the highest rates of opioid prescribing (Patrick et al. 2015) as well as in areas with higher rates of unemployment and shortages of mental health clinicians (Patrick et al. 2019).

The increase in opioid use among pregnant women is primarily attributed to increases in prescription opioid prescribing, with secondary waves of the opioid epidemic associated with illicit opioid use when prescription supplies were weaned through policy. Approximately 22–29% of pregnant women enrolled in public insurance and 14% of pregnant women enrolled in private insurance filled prescriptions for at least one opioid medication during their pregnancies (Bateman et al. 2014; Desai et al. 2015; Epstein et al. 2013). Women who are prescribed opioids or who have an opioid use disorder have high rates of co-occurring mental illness, including depression and anxiety (Arnaudo et al. 2017; Green et al. 2009; Holbrook and Kaltenbach 2012). Notably, pregnant women who use opioid medications are also more likely to be prescribed an SSRI and report higher rates of use of other substances, including tobacco, marijuana, and cocaine (American College of Obstetricians and Gynecologists 2017; Jones et al. 2009; Patrick et al. 2015).

As the opioid epidemic has progressed, there has been an increase in the treatment of opioid use disorder. Best practice treatments include medication-assisted treatment (MAT) with medications that also contain opioids (methadone or buprenorphine). Methadone has been the standard of care for treating pregnant women with opioid use disorder since the early 1990s, resulting in decreased opioid use among pregnant women. However, because methadone itself contains an opioid and because women receiving this treatment may have exposed their fetus to high levels of opioids before seeking treatment, methadone treatment has been associated with increased incidence of NAS and a longer duration of symptoms (Kaltenbach et al. 1998; Kandall et al. 1999). At Yale New Haven Children's Hospital (YNHCH), the number of infants exposed to methadone in utero increased by 74% over a 6-year period (2003–2009), and the average length of stay for infants with NAS following methadone exposure exceeded almost any other primary inpatient diagnoses (Grossman et al. 2017). Guidelines for the clinical use of buprenorphine with pregnant and postpartum women to treat opioid use disorder were released in 2015 (SAMHSA 2015). Buprenorphine has demonstrated similar efficacy as methadone in the treatment of opioid addiction during pregnancy, and there are some data suggesting buprenorphine may result in lower incidence and severity of NAS, reduced length of treatment, and better birth outcomes compared with methadone, although this research is limited (Brogly et al. 2014; Kocherlakota 2014).

Although the use of methadone and buprenorphine for the treatment of opioid use disorders during pregnancy is associated with NAS, the benefits of treatment for both mother and infant outweigh the risks. Women who receive these medication-assisted treatments for their opioid use disorder exhibit increased adherence to prenatal care and addiction treatment, reduced relapse risk, more stable fetal levels of opioids reducing risk for prenatal withdrawal, reduced rates of infectious disease (e.g., HIV, hepatitis C), improved birth outcomes compared to untreated pregnant women (e.g., gestational age, birth weight, lower risk for obstetric complications, and NAS), and greater numbers of infants in their mothers' care at 1 year of age

(American College of Obstetricians and Gynecologists 2017; Jones et al. 2008; Meyer et al. 2015).

1.3 Neurodevelopmental Outcomes Associated with NAS

Research on short- and long-term neurodevelopmental consequences of NAS is limited, and results are often confounded by environmental and social risk factors that are closely intertwined with substance use during pregnancy. However, for most infants with prenatal drug exposure, "the problems caused by maternal drug use do not stop during the neonatal period" (Oei 2019, p. 161 for quote) and are further complicated by intergenerational stressors like poverty, trauma exposure, malnutrition, and mental illness, which may compound any negative effect of direct drug exposure in utero.

Although the effects of direct substance exposure to the fetus are complicated by a multitude of factors, many substances have known teratogenic effects on fetal development. For example, opioids are known to impair neuronal development and function, and infants exposed to opioids in utero tend to have smaller head circumference and lower brain volumes, which has implications for cognitive development (Oei 2019). The literature also suggests that NAS may be associated with long-term outcomes such as general development, vision problems, motor issues, and behavioral and cognitive development (Maguire et al. 2016). Further, fetal substance exposure has also been associated with epigenetic changes that may increase later risk for developmental and behavioral problems (Chen et al. 2016).

However, the risks of direct substance exposure to the fetus are often exacerbated by lack of maternal healthcare access and utilization, including prenatal care. Mothers who use substances during pregnancy are at increased risk for chronic illnesses and infectious diseases that may negatively impact a pregnancy, as well as pregnancy and birth complications, including intrauterine growth restriction, uterine infection, maternal hypertension, placental abruption, preterm labor, low birth weight, miscarriage, and stillbirth (Sebastiani et al. 2018). Moreover, mothers who use substances during pregnancy are more likely to be homeless and experience food insecurity, which may lead to nutritional deficiencies, poor maternal weight gain, and, in turn, poor fetal growth and development (Sebastiani et al. 2018). Importantly, these pregnancy and birth complications are also associated with long-term developmental problems, making it difficult to parse the unique risks of fetal substance exposure from general maternal health and social status.

Paradoxically, risk for NAS increases with better birth outcomes, including good birth weight and term gestation, suggesting that with supportive care to resolve acute NAS symptoms, these infants may be able to retain a normal developmental trajectory (Hall et al. 2014). However, many of the risk factors associated with prenatal substance use continue to shape the early developmental environment, and there is a robust literature documenting the deleterious effects of poverty, family separation, parental mental illness, domestic violence, and neglect and maltreatment on infant and child development (Chartier et al. 2010; Dunn et al. 2002). These risks are exacerbated by broad societal inequalities, including racism and discrimination, inadequate healthcare and education, high rates of under- and unemployment, food insecurity, inadequate housing, and exposure to violence (Jansson and Velez 2012; Logan et al. 2013). Thus, NAS may be a downstream symptom or indicator of systemic social inequalities and intergenerational risk that heralds an opportunity to support the developmental trajectory of the infant through intervention on the system or, more specifically, the mother-infant dyad.

1.4 Assessment and Treatment of NAS

Neonatal outcomes including NAS symptom severity/duration, need for and length of pharmacotherapy, and length of hospital stay are important short-term markers of infant risk that reflect both individual and societal costs associated with prenatal substance exposure and NAS. Although these early consequences are not necessarily prognostic for infant health and functioning long term and it is short-sighted to focus on these outcomes separate from the broader social and developmental context, they provide important information about the course of the syndrome and the effectiveness of the supportive care and treatment provided to the infant and mother-infant dyad.

Infants exposed to substances during pregnancy are typically assessed and monitored for withdrawal symptoms beginning shortly after birth. Symptom screening tools like the Finnegan Neonatal Abstinence Scoring System (FNASS) are used to initiate and inform the course of treatment and determine the need for "supportive care" versus pharmacological intervention, continued hospitalization, or admission to the neonatal intensive care unit (NICU). Unfortunately, scoring systems like FNASS utilize arbitrary cutoff scores for initiation of pharmacotherapy and provide little information about the severity of symptoms or impacts on neonatal functioning, which would be most informative to guide treatment (Grisham et al. 2019; Grossman et al. 2018). Moreover, already fussy infants must be regularly disturbed to record FNASS information, which can exacerbate withdrawal symptoms (Grossman et al. 2018).

Methods of supportive care that have been shown to be beneficial for infants experiencing withdrawal symptoms include providing close relational experiences; swaddling; holding in arms; quiet, low-stimulation environment; small, "on-demand" feedings; waterbeds; and use of pacifiers. However, these approaches vary greatly in type and documented efficacy and are inconsistently implemented in the hospital setting (Clemans-Cope et al. 2020).

Pharmacological intervention to decrease withdrawal symptoms is required in 27% to 91% of infants with NAS (Greig et al. 2012; Kuschel 2007). Despite the significant number of infants requiring pharmacological intervention and the associated burden on healthcare expenditures, there is currently no uniformly accepted standardized regimen for the management of NAS symptoms (Hudak and Tan 2012). Kocherlakota's (2014) recent review recommends that pharmacological care be required only when (1) nonpharmacological interventions fail to improve NAS signs and symptoms, (2) withdrawal symptoms and severity persist, (3) critical symptoms are observed, and (4) acute dehydration follows vomiting and/or excessive diarrhea. However, administration of these guidelines is highly variable, and there are a range of inconsistent assessment strategies and medication regimens utilized to treat NAS.

Morphine is the most commonly used pharmacological approach to control severe NAS symptoms and decrease the incidence of seizures, diarrhea, agitation, and improve feeding (Jansson et al. 2009; Mehta et al. 2013; O'Grady et al. 2009). However, the dose of morphine, dependent on the severity of withdrawal symptoms, must be provided every 3–4 h, which requires consistent monitoring by a medical provider. An increasingly common pharmacological approach to the treatment of NAS is the use of methadone or buprenorphine, especially if the mothers were receiving MAT prenatally (Bio et al. 2011; Sarkar and Donn 2006). Although pharmacotherapy has allowed for the successful management of NAS symptoms, decreasing the likelihood of seizures and mortality for severely affected infants, it still has notable limitations (Newman et al. 2015).

Overall, pharmacological treatments require higher level of care that often prolong length of hospital stays and contribute to costly NICU hospitalizations. Infants requiring pharmacological treatment spend on average 23 days in the NICU, amounting to an average cost of $44,824 to $53,400 per infant with NAS (Grossman et al. 2017; Patrick et al. 2012). A paradox exists when treating NAS symptoms in the NICU. Infants appear to experience more severe NAS symptoms and exhibit a greater need for pharmacotherapy despite being in a more intensive treatment setting (Newman et al. 2015). Research from the Canadian Pediatric Society (2018) suggests that neither the NICU nor the pharmacological treatments may be necessary to treat NAS. Most infants with NAS are not critically ill or medically complex, meaning that they are taking up costly bed space in an unfavorable environment that poses barriers to parental caregiving and may inadvertently exacerbate NAS symptoms. NICUs also tend to be bustling environments that could overstimulate and irritate these infants and cause them to be more distressed and difficult to soothe (Grisham and Kane 2018). With NICU hospitalizations, infants are often separated from their mothers, and continuously monitored by nursing staff for symptoms, factors which may inadvertently lead to higher withdrawal scores and determination of the need for further pharmacotherapy (Vogel 2018). Notably, infants with NAS treated on general inpatient floors had 8.5-day average length of stay, compared with 23 days for infants in the NICU (Grossman et al. 2020).

Although it is recommended that supportive care and nonpharmacological methods be used as first-line interventions, the majority of infants with NAS are determined to require pharmacological interventions, suggesting that there is a great need to redefine standards of care as well as closely consider the goals of intervention to ensure there are agreed upon criteria for assessment and management of NAS, with a particular focus on the standardization of nonpharmacologic and pharmacologic interventions alike (Clemans-Cope et al. 2020). There are notable differences in the medical care administered as well as the potential long-term outcomes

Table 4.1 Comparing the standard treatment approach for NAS to family-centered care

Standard NAS treatment approach: focus on symptom suppression	Family-centered care for NAS: focus on promoting neonatal functioning
Medically-centered approach with emphasis on withdrawal symptoms	Family-centered approach with emphasis on supporting normal neonatal functioning, including developmental and relational needs
Focus is on withdrawal scores to determine need for treatment	Focus is on disruptions in normal neonatal functioning to determine need for treatment, specifically the ability to feed, sleep, and be consoled/soothed
Withdrawal scores do not differentiate types or severity of symptoms	
Medical providers administer care	Parents/caregivers administer care
Treatment focused on pharmacotherapy	Treatment focused on supportive care
Supportive care encouraged, but disrupted by assessment and treatment protocols	Pharmacotherapy as needed when withdrawal symptoms disrupt normal functioning despite supportive care
Parents/caregivers more likely to be separated from infants	Parents/caregivers and infants are kept together
	Parents/caregivers are considered "the treatment" and are expected/encouraged to administer care
Greater barriers to breastfeeding, skin-to-skin, and parental presence	Infants get more skin-to-skin, more likely to breastfeed
Parents/caregivers less involved in care and may experience difficult relationships with medical providers	Parents/caregivers coached on how to care for infants with special needs
More severe NAS symptoms	Less severe symptoms
Up to 98% infants receive pharmacotherapy	Decreased need for pharmacotherapy (10–15% of infants)
Require longer treatment with pharmacotherapy	Reduced length of treatment, hospitalization
Average length of stay: 23 days[a]	Average length of stay: 6 days[a]
Average cost of care: $44,824 per infant[a]	Average cost of care: $10,289 per infant[a]

Note. [a]Grossman et al. (2017).

when the primary goal of intervention or treatment is focused on *suppressing withdrawal symptoms* versus *promoting neonatal functioning* (Table 4.1). Even though nonpharmacological interventions are considered the first line of treatment, when the goal of care is symptom suppression, there tends to be a focus on the "medical needs" of the infant (versus developmental or relational needs), where emphasis is placed on withdrawal scores, leading to a tendency to treat the number. Additionally, when symptom suppression is the focus of treatment, pharmacotherapy may be considered the primary treatment tool; medical staff frequently take the lead in caregiving, with parents acting as supports or even spectators to caregiving; infants require longer and/or more intensive care; and "supportive care" including skin-to-skin contact, breastfeeding support, and other environmental or behavioral soothing techniques are often secondary to medical treatment (Grossman et al. 2018). The symptom-suppression approach to treatment can inadvertently alienate parents and promote contentious interactions with medical staff (Maguire et al. 2012) and often leads to more frequent or longer separations of infants from their mothers and family (Grisham and Kane 2018). Although this model of NAS care has been most common historically, in recent years, medical professionals and researchers alike advise that the weeks of separation involved in NAS treatment can be detrimental to early bonding and attachment (Newman et al. 2015; Vogel 2018) and, as previously mentioned, may paradoxically result in a more severe or chronic course of NAS (Grisham and Kane 2018).

In contrast, when the goal of NAS care is the promotion of normal neonatal functioning, the focus of care broadens to incorporate developmental and relational needs of the infant as key aspects of medical care, treating the whole infant and not just the NAS symptoms. Healthy bonding and attachment to caregivers is crucial for infant survival and development and is associated with long-term physical and social-emotional health (Crenshaw 2007). For example, early skin-to-skin contact is associated with larger head circumference at 8 weeks postpartum (Boo and Jamli 2007), and increased autonomic maturity (i.e., arousal regulation and increased shared attention) at 3 and 6 months postpartum, respectively (Feldman et al. 2002; Feldman and Eidelman 2003). Early opportunity to bond also stimulates the release of the hormone oxytocin, which promotes infant attachment, reduces stress, and helps support the infant during the postpartum transition (Buckley 2014; Crenshaw 2007; Moore et al. 2012). The release of oxytocin helps facilitate an infant's innate survival behaviors that lead to breastfeeding and behavioral regulation, whereas interrupting the initial attachment process can create difficulties for bonding and regulation over time (Crenshaw 2007).

1.5 Family-Centered Care for NAS

To develop healthy attachment, mothers and infants should be kept together and available to engage in unrestricted skin-to-skin contact and breastfeeding following birth (Crenshaw 2007), unless separation for medical reasons is warranted. Infants with NAS are more likely to be fussy as they are experiencing withdrawal symptoms, making a mother's undivided attention through consoling and feeding integral aspects of treatment (National Institute for Children's Health Quality 2020). Further, breastfeeding has been shown to decrease the need for pharmacological treatment and shorten the duration of NAS symptoms, consequently decreasing the length of hospital stay by 3–19 days (Abdel-Latif et al. 2007; Lefevere and Allegaert 2015; Pritham 2013). A recent study demonstrated that parental presence was associated with decreased NAS severity, decreased hospital stay length on average by 9 days, and reduced pharmacological treatment by 8 days (Howard et al. 2017). Studies have also shown skin-to-skin contact to be effective in managing NAS symptoms and to promote long-term functioning by improving infant sleep and autonomic nervous system function (Wu and Carre 2018).

Thus, promoting neonatal functioning means promoting a family-centered care approach (Fig. 4.1) in which mother and infant are kept together ("rooming-in");

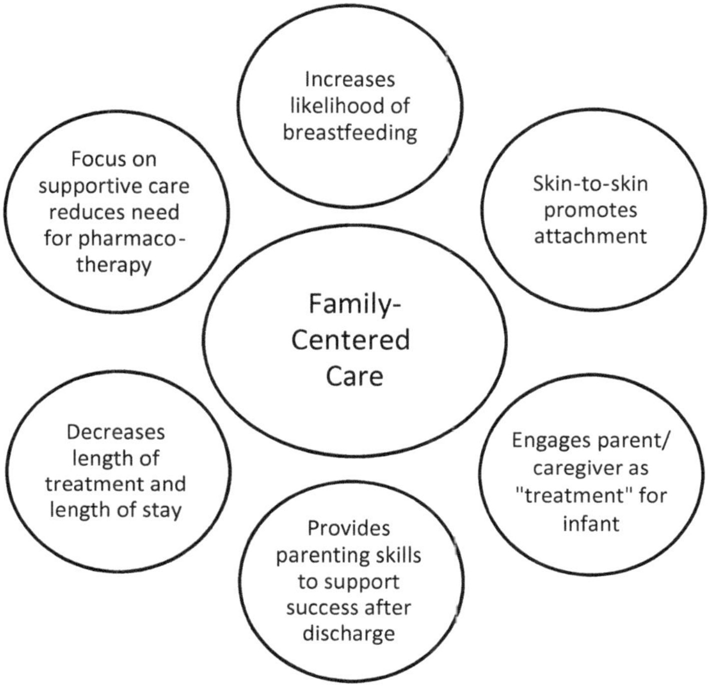

Fig. 4.1 Benefits of family-centered care

parents and parental caregiving become the primary treatment tool for administering supportive care, limiting interventions that irritate the infant and emphasizing skin-to-skin contact, breastfeeding support, and other soothing techniques as appropriate; medical providers partner with and coach parents on how to care for their infant and address acute and long-term needs; and medical interventions and pharmacotherapy are only utilized as necessary when infants show little improvement or worsening symptoms with only supportive care. Communication between medical providers and families is important for preparing families for NAS treatment and engaging them as part of the treatment team. To support family-centered care, medical providers are educated about addiction and trauma-informed care to reduce stigma and bias and are trained to interact non-judgmentally with families so that they feel valued and supported in caring for their infant (Atwood et al. 2016; Holmes et al. 2016).

Family-centered approaches like rooming-in and the Eat, Sleep, Console method (Grossman et al. 2018) have been shown to increase bonding and breastfeeding rates as well as reduce the length of hospital stays, NICU admissions, the use pharmacotherapy, and overall medical costs for opioid-exposed infants (Abrahams et al. 2007; Canadian Pediatric Society 2018; Holmes et al. 2016). More specifically, the Eat, Sleep, Console method (ESC; Grossman et al. 2018) empowers parents to be their infant's "treatment" by responding to their needs in the most naturalistic setting possible. ESC uses a functional scoring approach based on three key aspects of normal neonatal functioning to assess symptoms and guide NAS treatment: (1) Can the infant eat? (2) Can the infant sleep? and (3) Can the infant be consoled when distressed? (Grossman et al. 2018). Within this framework, infants are assessed on their ability to eat at least 1 oz. per bottle or breastfeed, their ability to sleep for at least 1 h undisturbed (may be in arms or with other environmental supports such as swaddling, swing, pacifier, etc.), and their ability to be consoled by their caregiver within 10 min (allows for another 10-min attempt with a second caregiver). If they are unable to eat due to distress, fatigue, or lack of coordination, providers may consider supplementing feedings with a nasogastric tube while continuing to support feedings by mouth. If infants are unable to sleep at least 1 h undisturbed or be consoled within 20 min due to excessive crying, motor movements, or other distress, providers may consider a one-time dose of morphine and reassess ESC after approximately 4 h. Additionally, assessments are completed in partnership with parents and importantly avoid disturbing the infant. Within this protocol, infants have unlimited access to bonding with caregivers, which is essential to both infant and parental mental health (Crenshaw 2007).

On average, 86% of mothers using the ESC method successfully breastfed their infants for 2.5 months, which is comparable to the US average of 83%, suggesting that the ESC helps facilitate positive parenting behaviors in a vulnerable population (Center for Disease Control 2018; Newman et al. 2015). Mothers who room-in with their infants (non-NAS sample) were found to spend more time looking at, talking to, and touching their infants (Prodromidis et al. 1995) and showed more affectionate behavior toward infants and "enhanced parenting" at a 17-month follow-up (O'Connor et al. 1980), behaviors that support and promote infant attachment and neurodevelopment (Crenshaw 2007).

Moreover, mothers themselves may demonstrate improved outcomes when they experience family-centered care and are able to room-in with their infants. There is evidence that family is a key motivator for substance abuse recovery. In particular, maintaining custody of and providing care to children may motivate substance use treatment and abstinence (see Villegas et al. 2016, for review), and in fact, mothers who roomed-in were more likely to retain custody of their children at discharge (Abrahams et al. 2007). Unfortunately, family-centered care for NAS is in its infancy, and there are currently no reports of longitudinal outcomes regarding parental substance use, parenting, risk for abuse or neglect, or infant neurodevelopment. However, an analysis of comprehensive residential substance abuse treatment programs that keep mothers and infants together suggests significant improvements in family functioning, including maintained recovery and abstinence (Porowski et al. 2004).

Considering short-term benefits associated with family-centered care, mothers and families are provided a protected opportunity to bond with their infant while learning to be attuned and responsive to their infant's unique needs. They have the opportunity to feel valued as a key component of the infant's care and treatment and have access to expert medical care and newborn care support to help them understand and ease their infant's withdrawal symptoms. Breastfeeding and skin-to-skin contact are associated with better maternal mental health (Bigelow et al. 2014), which is particularly important for mothers with substance use disorders who have an increased risk for overdose that peaks 7–12 months postpartum (Schiff et al. 2018). Mothers who roomed-in reported that they felt supported by medical providers and rated the experience favorably (Newman et al. 2015). Several mothers shared in qualitative responses that they appreciated the help and expertise of staff, that they felt supported and confident with the knowledge they gained, and that they felt fortunate to have the protected time for bonding with their infant (Newman et al. 2015). These findings suggest that family-centered care like rooming-in and the ESC method decrease infant stress and withdrawal symptoms while also empowering mothers from a historically stigmatized population. By reserving judgment and facilitating parenting behaviors, medical staff are able to empower mothers to be essential in NAS treatment, and help infants and their families to succeed following hospital discharge (Grossman et al. 2018) (Breakout Box 4.1).

Breakout Box 4.1. Focus on Practice

From my time as a pediatric resident, as well as my conversations with a number of NICU practitioners, it is clear to me that the relationship between a mother and her child is immeasurably powerful – not only in the setting of neonatal abstinence syndrome, but in all circumstances of life. Babies with attentive mothers who prioritize the mother-infant dyad tend to show less withdrawal symptoms, notably irritability, feeding problems, difficulty sleeping, and others. This decrease in symptoms undoubtedly results in a decrease in use of morphine and other pharmacologic treatment in many cases. The benefits of this bond are not limited to the baby; mothers with a history of substance abuse tend to have better outcomes themselves when their priorities are shifted towards their child. These mothers are often more motivated to seek treatment for substance abuse and are thus more likely to reach their goal of abstinence. Keeping this in mind, it is imperative to remove any stigma or bias that may be associated with this patient population. When treated not as an addict, but as a mother with promise and potential, feelings such as shame and worthlessness are eclipsed by feelings of purposefulness and commitment. As an osteopathic physician, a significant aspect of my training has been on emphasizing treatment of the patient, rather the disease – and I can think of no better way than to treat NAS using a family-centered approach when at all possible.

– Dr. Alexander Mach, D.O., Oklahoma State University/ Osteopathic Medical Education Consortium of Oklahoma Pediatric Resident.

1.6 Barriers to Family-Centered Care for NAS

Difficulties in accessing space, resources, and skilled staff to care for infants with NAS create unique barriers to family-centered care. One of the greatest challenges to the ESC model is having the space and resources to keep mothers and infants together (Vogel 2018). Some hospitals do not have the infrastructure or space to house the dyad in the same room and require unique problem solving to administer treatment. Grossman et al. (2018) describes one hospital's creative problem solving in closing off one area of NICU for more private, rooming-in treatment. Additionally, there is evidence that managing NAS care on general inpatient floors, rather than the NICU, reduces the use of pharmacotherapy and shortens the length of stay (Grossman et al. 2020), suggesting that hospitals may not require the creation of special accommodations for family-centered NAS treatment.

Another challenge to treatment is having nursing staff that feel confident working with mothers and families coping with substance use and addiction. Artigas (2017) suggests that some neonatal nurses feel moral distress related to treating infants with NAS whose mothers used illicit substances during pregnancy, which may contribute to lack of confidence or increased stress while working with infants with NAS (Vogel 2018) as well as strained interactions with parents (Maguire et al. 2012). Unfortunately, stigma and biases toward parents may have an unintended negative impact on the quality of nursing care (Raeside 2003), as well as possibly disrupt mother-infant bonding and impair infant outcomes (Marcellus 2014).

Substance use during pregnancy has been viewed as a public health and criminal justice issue, which has created stigma and barriers to care within the healthcare system (Stone 2015). Almost half of states in the United States have laws considering substance use during pregnancy as child abuse (Guttmacher Institute 2020), creating barriers for women seeking help, as well as legal and ethical dilemmas for providers and families. Although punitive policies may be created with the intention of deterring substance use during pregnancy and protecting infants, there is evidence that punitive policies are associated with increased rates of NAS (Faherty et al. 2019), suggesting such policies may actually exacerbate the risk for infants, possibly by discouraging women from seeking prenatal care and substance use treatment (Angelotta et al. 2016). Moreover, punitive policies increase the likelihood that infants will be separated from their mothers as well as increase the burden on child welfare and the foster care system, factors strongly associated with disrupted attachment and long-term developmental and social-emotional problems (Leslie et al. 2005). It is important to note that punitive policies may contribute to widening health inequality across class and race, as they disproportionately affect poor women and minorities who are more likely to utilize public health services, making them subject to increased surveillance, testing, and reporting (Paltrow and Flavin 2013; Stone 2015).

With evidence that these barriers and policies do little to improve outcomes associated with substance use during pregnancy and may actually result in poorer infant outcomes, there is a need to expand the implementation of evidence-informed approaches for the treatment of NAS like rooming-in and ESC, as well as increase the availability of and access to effective substance use treatment for pregnant and postpartum women (Faherty et al. 2019). Additionally, policies and programs that prevent and address the risk factors for substance use, including poverty, mental illness, trauma exposure, inadequate healthcare and education, and social inequalities, may serve to greatly reduce fetal substance exposure and promote the health and well-being of infants and their families (Stone 2015).

2 Implications

2.1 Implications for Understanding Family Resilience

Family-centered care, like ESC and rooming-in, focus on the family system, often the mother-infant dyad, to promote the infant's relational and developmental needs as integral aspects of medical treatment. This approach to healthcare creates family-provider partnerships that allow caregivers to be members of the medical team and engaged as equal team members throughout the medical decision-making process (Kuo et al. 2012). Although little outcome research exists on family-centered care for NAS, extant literature suggests that family-centered care models promote health literacy and medical self-management, as well as improve clinical decision making, factors that may foster collaborative interactions with medical providers and promote adherence and ongoing engagement with healthcare services (see Coulter and Ellins 2007, for a review; Kuo et al. 2012). Moreover, family-centered care has positive implications for parent and child well-being and overall family resilience (see Dunst et al. 2007, for a review).

Family-centered care models prioritize families' needs, culture, and dignity and aim to help families feel empowered as critical agents for wellness and recovery. Unfortunately, NAS can leave mothers feeling stigmatized within the healthcare system, and this bias toward caregivers may have unintended and unfortunate consequences for their infant's care (Raeside 2003). Family-centered care helps to reduce stigma as it emphasizes strength-based treatment and identifies parents and families as the experts of their own lived experiences whose contributions to care are crucial for the infants' recovery and long-term development success. In these models, medical providers receive training about substance use and trauma-informed care as well as how to curb stigma and bias in working with families coping with addiction. When mothers with substance use disorders are treated with dignity and are valued as members of the health care team, they become empowered to independently engage in caregiving behaviors, ultimately increasing the likelihood of success following hospital discharge (Abrahams et al. 2007; Grossman et al. 2018; Holmes et al. 2016).

Most importantly, family-centered care models, such as rooming-in and ESC, provide rich opportunities to improve the developmental trajectory for infants, compared to pharmacological NAS treatment. ESC emphasizes skin-to-skin contact, breastfeeding support, and soothing interventions, which are known to be associated with secure attachment, management of NAS symptoms, and reduced stress, promoting long-term functioning by improving infant sleep, autonomic nervous system function, and social-emotional health (Buckley 2014; Crenshaw 2007; Moore et al. 2012; Wu and Carre 2018).

Family-centered care interventions also have benefits for mothers and families. Breastfeeding and skin-to-skin contact, essential components of ESC and nonpharmacological interventions for NAS, reduce the risk for maternal depression and anxiety symptoms, which is particularly important for mothers with substance use disorders who have an increased risk for mental illness and overdose in the postpartum (Schiff et al. 2018). With the support of family-centered care approaches, mothers are able to focus on their infant's and family's well-being, which is known motivator in substance use recovery (Villegas et al. 2016). Healthcare professionals help foster resilience within parents and families as they coach caregivers in caring for fussy infants, addressing withdrawal symptoms, and responding to their infants' cues, skills that both help to reduce NAS symptoms and promote attachment and infant neurodevelopment (Crenshaw 2007; Vogel 2018). Moreover, as infants are less likely to be separated from caregivers during treatment and at hospital discharge (Abrahams et al. 2007), these family-centered approaches may reduce the risks for ongoing adverse experiences and the transmission of intergenerational trauma, boost family resilience, and help to keep families together long term.

2.2 *Implications for Practice and/or Policy*

In order to implement the most effective and comprehensive plan of care for each family, programs should implement a multidisciplinary approach, where all professionals including counselors, social workers, healthcare providers, and legal system professionals take an active role (SAMHSA 2016). Importantly, every professional involved should be trained in evidence-based care practices, risks associated with substance use during pregnancy, and factors that promote optimal infant and family functioning (US Department of Health and Human Services, Health Resources and Services Administration (HRSA) 2018). Women who use substances during pregnancy face many barriers to care, and in particular, many women fear that seeking prenatal care and substance use treatment during pregnancy will lead to criminalization and social stigma (Ecker et al. 2019). Thus, to promote long-term resilience and positive outcomes for infants and children, policies and practices should aim to develop strategies that promote the health, safety, well-being, and recovery of pregnant women with opioid use disorders and their infants, while nonjudgmentally respecting their ability to care for their infants, so that they are able to develop the skills and have the support they need to be successful.

Further, it is imperative that practice and policies utilize state- and community-level strategies to gain access to space, resources, and skilled staff to care for infants with NAS. Specifically, there is a need to expand the implementation of evidence-informed approaches for the assessment and treatment of NAS, particularly family-centered models, as well as increase the availability of and access to effective substance use screening and treatment for pregnant and postpartum women (Faherty et al. 2019; Grossman et al. 2018). For example, to help bolster long-term success following discharge, mothers should retain access to healthcare services, including continued support for substance use treatment, which may include a combination of pharmacotherapy, behavioral interventions, and psychiatric care. Further, mothers may benefit from education related to their infant's behaviors and attachment, and intensive support services, including developmental guidance and early childhood intervention services (Grossman et al. 2018; SAMHSA 2016).

Moreover, public health approaches should begin by prioritizing the standardization, affordability, and accessibility of primary prevention strategies, including routine physical and behavioral healthcare, family planning and reproductive services, and responsible opioid prescribing (see Faherty et al. 2019). Additionally, it is recommended that screening for substance use be incorporated as a critical component of comprehensive obstetric care that collaboratively occurs during routine prenatal care appointments (ACOG 2017). Early *universal* screening, such as the National Institute on Drug Abuse (NIDA) Quick Screen Tool, alongside brief intervention and treatment referral information, is important for reducing biases and related stigma, while also promoting long-term maternal and infant health outcomes (ACOG 2017; Ecker et al. 2019). Importantly, professionals and pregnant women alike should understand the implications and the interventions most effective for treating substance use during the prenatal and postpartum period, and women should be active participants in the decision-making process about their care (Ecker et al. 2019).

Given that some professionals experience moral distress, lack of confidence, and increased stress when working with substance-exposed infants and mothers who use/used substances during pregnancy, it may be imperative to provide additional education and support to professionals (Artigas 2017; Maguire et al. 2012; Vogel 2018). For example, specialized training in addiction medicine and substance use treatment is important for increasing professionals' education and confidence, decreasing stress levels, and ultimately improving patient-provider interactions (Cleveland and Gill 2013). Additionally, adopting a trauma-informed approach to care is one way to teach professionals how to recognize and help families respond to the effects of adversity that often accompany substance use (HRSA 2018). Further, reflective supervision could serve as an additional support tool for professionals to collaboratively reflect on the emotional work of patient-provider interactions (HRSA 2018). In fact, there is evidence to suggest that training providers in trauma-informed approaches, while supporting them through reflective supervision, is an effective strategy to helping pregnant women and caregivers best care for their infants (HRSA 2018). Importantly, these strategies help to promote a compassionate approach among professionals to ensure practice is being conducted in a manner that respects the dignity of all caregivers and minimizes biases, while also balancing social expectations and family safety (Johnson 2017).

Importantly, there is strong evidence that family-centered treatment for NAS is associated with significantly reduced hospital costs, a function of reductions in the use of pharmacological treatment, reduced lengths of stay for NAS treatment, and reduced NICU utilization (Holmes et al. 2016). This has particularly important implications for public health costs and taxpayer-funded programs like public health insurance options (i.e., Medicaid), as the incidence of NAS was found to be over 7 times higher among infants covered by public health insurance, along with longer lengths of stay and higher rates of hospital transfers, compared to infants with private insurance coverage (Winkelman et al. 2018). Winkelman et al. (2018) point out that the Centers for Medicare and Medicaid Services and state Medicaid programs, as the leading payers of NAS-related care in the United States, have the ability and opportunity to set national standards for NAS-related care that addresses the "triple aim" of reduced costs, improved outcomes, and enhanced experiences for infants and families (Berwick et al. 2008; Patrick 2015). As noted in this review, the systematic implementation of family-centered care protocols in various hospital systems has demonstrated striking results in regard to improved outcomes, reduced costs and improved experiences for families (Atwood et al. 2016), and likely has significant potential to promote infant attachment and parental bonding. Thus, the standardization and widespread implementation of family-centered care for NAS should be considered a top priority by public health agencies and insurance payers who aim to improve maternal and infant outcomes while reducing costs (Winkelman et al. 2018).

Finally, practice and policies should also aim to address the risk factors for substance use, including poverty, mental illness, trauma exposure, inadequate healthcare and education, and social inequalities, because this may serve to greatly reduce fetal substance exposure and promote the health and well-being of infants and their families (Stein et al. 2017). In fact, research suggests that systems-level approaches indirectly addressing substance use are most effective at preventing negative health and social consequences associated with addiction (SAMHSA 2016). Specifically, family-centered and gender-responsive approaches, including prolonged, multidisciplinary interventions that aim to keep mothers and their infant together, have been shown to demonstrate positive and cost-effective outcomes and, thus, should be made more available and accessible (Abrahams et al. 2007; Canadian Pediatric Society 2018; Holmes et al. 2016).

3 Conclusion and Future Directions

Family-centered approaches and treatment programs that keep mothers and infants together may be key to reducing morbidity and improving long-term outcomes for substance-exposed infants and their families. Early research suggests that approaches like ESC and rooming-in are effective and even superior to standard NAS care in terms of short-term outcomes for infants, including reduced need for pharmacotherapy, less severe and shorter duration of withdrawal symptoms, less intensive treatment environments, shorter hospitalizations, and significantly reduced costs. Moreover, there is evidence from the literatures on attachment, substance use treatment, and family-centered care that these approaches may have long-term benefits for infants, mothers, and families alike, including improved neurodevelopment, adherence to substance use treatment, positive engagement with the healthcare system, positive parenting practices, reduced risk for adversity, and improved family functioning and resilience. However, much more research is needed to determine whether these long-term benefits are seen with infants with NAS who received family-centered care (compared to standard pharmacological treatment), as currently no longitudinal studies exist that examine outcomes post-discharge (Grossman et al. 2018).

More specifically, the field would benefit from future research that examines infant functioning following discharge, including health and developmental outcomes like growth, cognitive and language development, social-emotional development, and attachment, to determine whether family-centered care for NAS is associated with improved outcomes compared to infants with NAS who received more standard treatment. Additional outcomes assessing the quality of parental caregiving, parental mental health, parental substance use, and overall family functioning are important for understanding the effect of NAS treatment on the family system, which itself has major implications for infant outcomes long term. Importantly, there is a need to standardize family-centered NAS treatment protocols as well as determine the critical components of care, that is, the primary mechanisms that drive the improvement in outcomes. For example, it is important to determine whether it is the consumption of breast milk alone or the experience of being breastfed by the mother that drives the reduction in NAS symptoms; or whether additional parental preparation and coaching about NAS and infant behavior improves infant outcomes over and above parental presence alone. Finally, establishing a standard implementation plan for other hospitals and medical centers to adopt family-centered care practices for NAS would be helpful in expanding the availability to diverse communities and examining individual differences in treatment outcomes. Although much more information is needed on family-centered care for NAS, it is clear that this is a promising treatment approach that has great potential to create change in the family system and infants' developmental trajectories.

Acknowledgment This work was supported through the Center for Integrated Research on Child Adversity (CIRCA) and the National Institute of General Medical Sciences (NIGMS) of the National Institutes of Health under Award Number P20GM109097.

Glossary of Terms

Early Universal Screening Screening tool or assessment used to identify at risk individuals to help with prevention of a particular disorder.

Eat, Sleep, Console (ESC) Method A family-centered model of treatment that focuses on the comfort and care of infants at risk for NAS by maximizing non-pharmacologic intervention and increasing family involvement in treatment.

Family Centered Care Care aimed at developing and maintaining the family's role in a collaborative way with the clinical care team (such as nurses and doctors). This type of care views the entire family as the patient, not just the infant.

Finnegan Neonatal Abstinence Scoring System (FNASS) Symptom screening tool that assesses 21 of the most common signs of NAS, which are scored on the basis of pathological significance and severity to determine initiation of pharmacotherapy.

Illicit Drug Illegal substances that either stimulate or inhibit the central nervous system or cause hallucinogenic effects.

In Utero Latin for "in the womb" or "in the uterus".

Infant Attachment The emotional connection that an infant forms with their caregiver(s). Attachment is characterized by an infant's inclination to seek and maintain closeness to their caregiver(s), especially during stressful situations.

Intergenerational Stressors Stressors such as poverty, trauma exposure, malnutrition, and mental illness that occur in families over multiple generations.

Medication-Assisted Therapy (MAT) Type of substance use treatment that combines the use of medications, such as methadone or buprenorphine, with behavioral therapy techniques.

Nasogastric Tube A tube that is passed through the nose and the esophagus to carry food or medicine down into a patient's stomach.

Neonatal Period when infant is a newborn.

Neonatal Abstinence Syndrome (NAS) Complex syndrome that is characterized by signs and symptoms of substance withdrawal with an infant, primarily involving the central and autonomic nervous systems and the gastrointestinal system.

Neonatal Intensive Care Unit (NICU) A nursery in a hospital that provides intensive care to ill, medically-fragile, or premature infants.

Opioid Class of drug naturally found in the opium poppy plant. Examples include heroin, fentanyl, and prescription opioids such as Vicodin and OxyContin.

Opioid Agonist Treatment (also Opioid Substitution Program) Treatment for opioid addiction that involves taking opioid agonists such as methadone or buprenorphine.

Pharmacotherapy Type of medical treatment by means of drugs such as methadone and buprenorphine.

Punitive Policies Policies that are intended to punish individuals for their actions and remove them from society through incarceration.

Rooming-In Evidence-based practice that encourages keeping newborn infants and their mothers together in post-labor recovery rooms.

Selective Serotonin Reuptake Inhibitors (SSRIs) Class of antidepressant medication that is most commonly used.

Substance Use Disorder Occurs when an individual's use of a substance leads to health difficulties or issues at home, work, or school.

Teratogenic Effects An effect caused by a drug, chemical, or infection during pregnancy that resulted in a birth defect.

Tricyclic Antidepressants (TCAs) Class of antidepressant medication.

Withdrawal The onset of symptoms (physical and mental) when a substance is reduced or not given to the body.

Questions for Thought and Discussion

1. The use of opioid-substitution programs has increased with the treatment of opioid use during pregnancy, but comes with its own disadvantages. What are the advantages and disadvantages of these programs?
2. Family-centered care can be used as a primary treatment for NAS. How does family-centered care differ from other treatment models, and what are its benefits?
3. When it comes to the treatment of NAS, why is it important for the family and healthcare providers (such as nurses and doctors) to collaborate on treatment and care for the infant?
4. Why might the assessment of implicit biases and stigma be important for providers working with infants with NAS, and their families?
5. Discuss the benefits of approaching treatment of NAS with the goal of *promoting neonatal functioning*, as compared to *suppressing withdrawal symptoms*.
6. Propose a research study to examine the outcomes of the Eat, Sleep, Console method?
7. What are the benefits of early universal screening? In what ways does early universal screening reduce biases and related stigma?
8. Discuss the ways the following factors may increase risk for substance use: poverty, mental illness, trauma exposure, inadequate healthcare and education, and social inequalities.
9. Discuss the ways punitive policies that criminalize substance use during pregnancy may be detrimental to the infants they were designed to protect?
10. Clinical scenario: A pregnant woman seeks treatment for her misuse of prescribed medications, including benzodiazepines, amphetamines, or other pharmacotherapies, and wants to receive care that would best protect her health and the health of her fetus (SAMHSA 2016, 2018). Discuss a possible course of treatment and the providers involved.

References

Abdel-Latif, M. E., Bajuk, B., Lui, K., Oei, J., & NSW on ACT Neonatal Intensive Care Units' Study (NICUS) Group. (2007). Short-term outcomes of infants of substance-using mothers admitted to neonatal intensive care units in New South Wales and the Australian Capital Territory. *Journal of Paediatrics and Child Health, 43*(3), 127–133. https://doi.org/10.1111/j.1440-1754.2007.01031.x.

Abrahams, R. R., Kelly, S. A., Payne, S., Thiessen, P. N., Mackintosh, J., & Janssen, P. A. (2007). Rooming-in compared with standard care for newborns of mothers using methadone or heroin. *Canadian Family Physician, 53*(10), 1722–1730.

American College of Obstetricians and Gynecologists. (2017). *ACOG Committee Opinion, Number 711. Opioid use and opioid use disorder in pregnancy*. American College of Obstetrics and Gynecologists. Retrieved from https://www.acog.org/clinical/clinical-guidance/committee-opinion/articles/2017/08/opioid-use-and-opioid-use-disorder-in-pregnancy

Angelotta, C., Weiss, C. J., Angelotta, J. W., & Friedman, R. A. (2016). A moral or medical problem: The relationship between legal penalties and treatment practices for opioid use disorders in pregnant women. *Women's Health Issues, 26*(6), 595–601. https://doi.org/10.1016/j.whi.2016.09.002.

Arnaudo, C. L., Andraka-Christou, B., & Allgood, K. (2017). Psychiatric co-morbidities in pregnant women with opioid use disorders: Prevalence, impact, and implications for treatment. *Current Addiction Reports, 4*(1), 1–13. https://doi.org/10.1007/s40429-017-0132-4.

Artigas, V. (2017). *Do neonatal nurses caring for newborns with neonatal abstinence syndrome (NAS) whose mothers used illicit substances during pregnancy experience moral distress? A pilot study*. (Unpublished Doctoral Dissertation). University of Connecticut, Connecticut. Retrieved from https://opencommons.uconn.edu/dissertations/1677

Atwood, E. C., Sollender, G., Hsu, E., Arsnow, C., Flanagan, V., Celenza, J., Whalen, B., & Holmes, A. V. (2016). A qualitative study of family experience with hospitalization for neonatal abstinence syndrome. *Hospital Pediatrics, 6*(10), 626–632. https://doi.org/10.1542/hpeds.2016-0024.

Banta-Green, C. J., Merrill, J. O., Doyle, S. R., Boudreau, D. M., & Calsyn, D. A. (2009). Opioid use behaviors, mental health and pain – Development of a typology of chronic pain patients. *Drug and Alcohol Dependence, 104*(1–2), 34–42. https://doi.org/10.1016/j.drugalcdep.2009.03.021.

Bateman, B. T., Hernandez-Diaz, S., Rathmell, J. P., Seeger, J. D., Doherty, M., Fischer, M. A., & Huybrechts, K. F. (2014). Patterns of opioid utilization in pregnancy in a large cohort of commercial insurance beneficiaries in the United States. *Anesthesiology, 120*(5), 1216–1224. https://doi.org/10.1097/aln.0000000000000172.

Berwick, D. M., Nolan, T. W., & Whittington, J. (2008). The triple aim: Care, health, and cost. *Health Affairs, 27*, 759–769. https://doi.org/10.1377/hlthaff.27.3.759.

Bigelow, A. E., Power, M., Gillis, D. E., Maclellan-Peters, J., Alex, M., & McDonald, C. (2014). Breastfeeding, skin-to-skin contact, and mother-infant interactions over infants' first three months. *Infant Mental Health Journal, 35*(1), 51–62. https://doi.org/10.1002/imhj.21424.

Bio, L. L., Siu, A., & Poon, C. Y. (2011). Update on the pharmacologic management of neonatal abstinence syndrome. *Journal of Perinatology, 31*(11), 692–701. https://doi.org/10.1038/jp.2011.116.

Boo, N. Y., & Jamli, F. M. (2007). Short duration of skin-to-skin contact: Effects on growth and breastfeeding. *Journal of Paediatrics and Child Health, 43*(12), 831–836. https://doi.org/10.1111/j.1440-1754.2007.01198.x.

Brogly, S. B., Saia, K. A., Walley, A. Y., Du, H. M., & Sebastiani, P. (2014). Prenatal buprenorphine versus methadone exposure and neonatal outcomes: Systematic review and meta-analysis. *American Journal of Epidemiology, 180*(7), 673–686. https://doi.org/10.1093/aje/kwu190.

Buckley, S. J. (2014). *The hormonal physiology of childbearing*. New York: Childbirth Connection.

Canadian Pediatric Society. (2018). *Managing infants born to mothers who have used opioids during pregnancy*. Retrieved from https://www.cps.ca/en/documents/position/opioids-during-pregnancy.

Center for Behavioral Health Statistics and Quality (CBHSQ). (2018). *2017 National survey on drug use and health.* Rockville: Substance Abuse and Mental Health Services Administration. Retrieved from https://www.samhsa.gov/data/release/2017-national-survey-drug-use-and-health-nsduh-releases

Center for Disease Control. (2018). *Breastfeeding report card.* Retrieved from https://www.cdc.gov/breastfeeding/data/reportcard.htm

Centers for Disease Control and Prevention. (2020). *Data and statistics about opioid use during pregnancy*. Retrieved from https://www.cdc.gov/pregnancy/opioids/data.html#:~:text=Neonatal%20Abstinence%20Syndrome%20(NAS)&text=That%20is%20approximately%20one%20baby,80%20newborns%20diagnosed%20every%20day

Chartier, M. J., Walker, J. R., & Naimark, B. (2010). Separate and cumulative effects of adverse childhood experiences in predicting adult health and health care utilization. *Child Abuse and Neglect, 34*(6), 454–464. https://doi.org/10.1016/j.chiabu.2009.09.020.

Chen, Q., Yan, W., & Duan, E. (2016). Epigenetic inheritance of acquired traits through sperm RNAs and sperm RNA modifications. *Nature Reviews Genetics, 17*(12), 733–743. https://doi.org/10.1038/nrg.2016.106.

Clemans-Cope, L., Holla, N., Lee, H. C., Cong, A. S., Castro, R., Chyi, L., Huang, A., Taylor, K. J., & Kenney, G. M. (2020). Neonatal abstinence syndrome management in California birth hospitals: Results of a statewide survey. *Journal of Perinatology, 40*, 463–472. https://doi.org/10.1038/s41372-019-0568-6.

Cleveland, L. M. & Gill, S. L. (2013). "Try not to judge": Mothers of substance exposed infants. *The American Journal of Maternal/Child Nursing, 38*(4), 200–205. https://doi.org/10.1097/NMC.0b013e31827816de

Crenshaw, J. T. (2007). Health baby practices #6: Keep mother and baby together – It's best for mother, baby, and breastfeeding. *The Journal of Perinatal Education, 23*(4), 211–217. https://doi.org/10.1891/1058-1243.23.4.211.

Coulter, A. & Ellins, J. (2007). Effectiveness of strategies for informing, educating, and involving patients. *British Medical Journal, 335*(24), 24–27. https://doi.org/10.1136/bmj.39246.581169.80

Desai, R. J., Huybrechts, K. F., Hernandez-Diaz, S., Mogun, H., Patorno, E., Kaltenbach, K., Kerzner, L. S., & Bateman, B. T. (2015). Exposure to prescription opioid analgesics in utero and risk of neonatal abstinence syndrome: Population based cohort study. *BMJ, 350*, h2102. https://doi.org/10.1136/bmj.h2102.

Dunn, M. G., Tarter, R. E., Mezzich, A. C., Vanyukov, M., Kirisci, L., & Kirillova, G. (2002). Origins and consequences of child neglect in substance abuse families. *Clinical Psychology Review, 22*, 1063–1090. https://doi.org/10.1016/S0272-7358(02)00132-0.

Dunst, C. J., Trivette, C. M., & Hamby, D. W. (2007). Meta-analysis of family-centered helpgiving practices research. *Mental Retardation and Developmental Disabilities Research Reviews, 13*, 370–378. https://doi.org/10.1002/mrdd.20176

Ecker, J., Abuhamed A., Hill, W., Bailit, J., Bateman, B. T., Berghella, V., ... & Yonkers, K. A. (2019). Substance use disorders in pregnancy: Clinical, ethical, and research imperatives of the opioid epidemic: A report of a joint workshop of the Society for Maternal-Fetal Medicine, American College of Obstetricians, and Gynecologists, and American Society of Addiction Medicine. *Society for Maternal-Fetal Medicine, 221*(1), 5–28. https://doi.org/10.1016/j.ajog.2019.03.022

Epstein, R. A., Bobo, W. V., Martin, P. R., Morrow, J. A., Wang, W., Chandrasekhar, R., & Cooper, W. O. (2013). Increasing pregnancy-related use of prescribed opioid analgesics. *Annals of Epidemiology, 23*(8), 498–503. https://doi.org/10.1016/j.annepidem.2013.05.017.

Faherty, L. J., Kranz, A. M., Russell-Fritch, J., Patrick, S. W., Cantor, J., & Stein, B. D. (2019). Association of punitive and reporting state policies related to substance use in pregnancy with rates of neonatal abstinence syndrome. *JAMA Network Open, 2*(11), e1914078. https://doi.org/10.1001/jamanetworkopen.2019.14078.

Feldman, R., & Eidelman, A. I. (2003). Skin-to-skin contact (Kangaroo care) accelerates autonomic and neurobehavioural maturation in preterm infants. *Developmental Medicine and Child Neurology, 45*, 274–281. https://doi.org/10.1017/s0012162203000525.

Feldman, R., Weller, A., Sirota, L., & Eidelman, A. I. (2002). Skin-to-skin contact (Kangaroo care) promotes self-regulation in premature infants: Sleep-wake cyclicity, arousal modulation, and sustained exploration. *Developmental Psychology, 38*(2), 194–207. https://doi.org/10.1037/0012-1649.38.2.194.

Greig, E., Ash, A., & Douiri, A. (2012). Maternal and neonatal outcomes following methadone substitution during pregnancy. *Archives of Gynecology and Obstetrics, 286*(4), 843–851. https://doi.org/10.1007/s00404-012-2372-9.

Grisham, L., & Kane, M. (2018). A new approach to NAS – Home in six days [Powerpoint Slides]. Retrieved from http://www.nationalperinatal.org/resources/Documents/2018%20Conference/Thursday/A3%20-%20Grisham%20and%20Kane%20%20A%20New%20Approach%20to%20NAS%20-%20Home%20in%20Six%20Days_NPA.pdf

Grisham, L. M., Stephen, M. M., Coykendall, M. R., Kane, M. F., Maurer, J. A., & Bader, M. Y. (2019). Eat, sleep, console approach: A family-centered model for the treatment of neonatal abstinence syndrome. *Advances in Neonatal Care, 19*(2), 138–144. https://doi.org/10.1097/anc.0000000000000581.

Grossman, M. R., Berkwitt, A. K., Osborn, R. R., Xu, Y., Esserman, D. A., Shapiro, E. D., & Bizzarro, M. J. (2017). An initiative to improve the quality of care of infants with neonatal abstinence syndrome. *Pediatrics, 139*(6), e20163360. https://doi.org/10.1542/peds.2016-3360.

Grossman, M. R., Lipshaw, M. J., Osborn, R. R., & Berkwitt, A. K. (2018). A novel approach to assessing infants with neonatal abstinence syndrome. *Hospital Pediatrics, 8*(1), 1–6. https://doi.org/10.1542/hpeds.2017-0128.

Grossman, M. R., Berkwitt, A. K., Osborn, R. R., Citarella, B. V., Hochreiter, D., & Bizzarro, M. J. (2020). Evaluating the effect of hospital setting on outcomes for neonatal abstinence syndrome. *Journal of Perinatology*. https://doi.org/10.1038/s41372-020-0621-5.

Guttmacher Institute. (2020). *Substance use during pregnancy*. https://www.guttmacher.org/state-policy/explore/substance-use-during-pregnancy

Haight, S. C., Ko, J. Y., Tong, V. T., Bohm, M. K., & Callaghan, W. M. (2018). Opioid use disorder documented at delivery hospitalization – United States, 1999–2014. *Morbidity and Mortality Weekly Report, 67*(31), 845–849. https://doi.org/10.15585/mmwr.mm6731a1.

Hall, E. S., Wexelblatt, S. L., Crowley, M., Grow, J. L., Jasin, L. R., Klebanoff, M. A., McClead, R. E., Meinzen-Derr, J., Mohan, V. K., Stein, H., Walsh, M. C., & OCHNAS Consortium. (2014). A multicenter cohort study of treatments and hospital outcomes in neonatal abstinence syndrome. *Pediatrics, 134*(2), e527–e534. https://doi.org/10.1542/peds.2013-4036.

Health Resources and Services Administration (HRSA). (2018). *Substance use disorders and primary care integration*. Retrieved from https://bphc.hrsa.gov/qualityimprovement/clinicalquality/substance-use-disorder-primary-care-integration

Holbrook, A., & Kaltenbach, K. (2012). Co-occurring psychiatric symptoms in opioid-dependent women: The prevalence of antenatal and postnatal depression. *The American Journal of Drug and Alcohol Abuse, 38*(6), 575–579. https://doi.org/10.3109/00952990.2012.696168.

Holmes, A. V., Atwood, E. C., Whalen, B., Beliveau, J., Jarvis, D., Matulis, J. C., & Ralston, S. L. (2016). Rooming-in to treat neonatal abstinence syndrome: Improved family-centered care at lower cost. *Pediatrics, 137*(6), e20152929. https://doi.org/10.1542/peds.2015-2929.

Howard, M. B., Schiff, D. M., Penwill, N., Si, W., Rai, A., Wolfgang, T., Moses, J. M., & Wachman, E. W. (2017). Impact of parental presence at infants' bedside on neonatal abstinence syndrome. *Hospital Pediatrics, 7*(2), 63–69. https://doi.org/10.1542/hpeds.2016-0147

Hudak, M. L., & Tan, R. C. (2012). Neonatal drug withdrawal. *Pediatrics, 129*(2), e540–e560. https://doi.org/10.1542/peds.2011-3212.

Jansson, L. M., & Velez, M. (2012). Neonatal abstinence syndrome. *Current Opinion in Pediatrics, 24*(2), 252–258. https://doi.org/10.1097/mop.0b013e32834fdc3a.

Jansson, L. M., Velez, M., & Harrow, C. (2009). The opioid exposed newborn: Assessment and pharmacologic management. *Journal of Opioid Management, 5*(1), 47–55.

Johnson, R. F. (2017). Going beyond 'do no harm': A critical annotation. *Annals of Palliative Medicine, 6*(2), 266–268. https://doi.org/10.21037/apm.2017.09.08

Jones, H. E., O'Grady, K. E., Malfi, D., & Tuten, M. (2008). Methadone maintenance vs. methadone taper during pregnancy: Maternal and neonatal outcomes. *The American Journal on Addictions, 17*(5), 372–386. https://doi.org/10.1080/10550490802266276.

Jones, H. E., Heil, S. H., O'Grady, K. E., Martin, P. R., Kaltenbach, K., Coyle, M. G., … & Fischer, G. (2009). Smoking in pregnant women screened for an opioid agonist medication study compared to related pregnant and non-pregnant patient samples. The American Journal of Drug and Alcohol Abuse, 35(5), 375–380. doi:https://doi.org/10.1080/00952990903125235.

Kaltenbach, K., Berghella, V., & Finnegan, L. (1998). Opioid dependence during pregnancy: Effects and management. *Obstetrics and Gynecology Clinics of North America, 25*(1), 139–151. https://doi.org/10.1016/s0889-8545(05)70362-4.

Kandall, S. R., Doberczak, T. M., Jantunen, M., & Stein, J. (1999). The methadone-maintained pregnancy. *Clinics in Perinatology, 26*(1), 173–183. https://doi.org/10.1016/S0095-5108(18)30077-0.

Kocherlakota, P. (2014). Neonatal abstinence syndrome. *Pediatrics, 134*(2), 547–561. https://doi.org/10.1542/peds.2013-3524.

Kuo, D. Z., Houtrow, A. J., Arango, P., Kuhlthau, K. A., Simmons, J. M., & Neff, J. M. (2012). Family-centered care: Current applications and future directions in pediatric health care. *Maternal and Child Health Journal, 16*, 297–305. https://doi.org/10.1007/s10995-011-0751-7

Kuschel, C. (2007). Managing drug withdrawal in the newborn infant. *Seminars in Fetal & Neonatal Medicine, 12*(2), 127–133. https://doi.org/10.1016/j.siny.2007.01.004.

Lefevere, J. & Allegaert, K. (2015). Is breastfeeding useful in the management of neonatal abstinence syndrome? *Archives of Disease in Childhood, 100*(4), 414–415. https://doi.org/10.1136/archdischild-2015-308275

Leslie, L. K., Gordon, J. N., Lambros, K., Premji, K., Peoples, J., & Gist, K. (2005). Addressing the developmental and mental health needs of young children in foster care. *Journal of Developmental & Behavioral Pediatrics, 26*(2), 140–151. https://doi.org/10.1097/00004703-200504000-00011.

Logan, B. A., Brown, M. S., & Hayes, M. J. (2013). Neonatal abstinence syndrome: Treatment and pediatric outcomes. *Clinical Obstetrics and Gynecology, 56*(1), 186–192. https://doi.org/10.1097/grf.0b013e31827feea4.

Maguire, D., Webb, M., Passmore, D., & Cline, G. (2012). NICU nurse's lived experience: Caring for infants with neonatal abstinence syndrome. *Advances in Neonatal Care, 12*, 281–285. https://doi.org/10.1097/ANC.0b013e3182677bc1.

Maguire, D. J., Taylor, S., Armstrong, K., Shaffer-Hudkins, E., Germain, A. M., Brooks, S. S., Cline, G. J., & Clark, L. (2016). Long-term outcomes of infants with neonatal abstinence syndrome. *Neonatal Network, 35*(5), 277–286. https://doi.org/10.1891/0730-0832.35.5.277.

Marcellus, L. (2014). Supporting women with substance use issues: Trauma-informed care as a foundation for practice in the NICU. *Neonatal Network, 33*, 307–314. https://doi.org/10.1891/0730-0832.33.6.307.

Martin, C. E., Longinaker, N., & Terplan, M. (2015). Recent trends in treatment admissions for prescription opioid abuse during pregnancy. *Journal of Substance Abuse Treatment, 48*(1), 37–42. https://doi.org/10.1016/j.jsat.2014.07.007.

McQueen, K., & Murphy-Oikonen, J. (2016). Neonatal abstinence syndrome. *New England Journal of Medicine, 375*(25), 2468–2479. https://doi.org/10.1056/nejmra1600879.

Mehta, A., Forbes, K. D., & Kuppala, V. S. (2013). Neonatal abstinence syndrome management from prenatal counseling to postdischarge follow-up care: Results of a national survey. *Hospital Pediatrics, 3*(4), 317–323. https://doi.org/10.1542/hpeds.2012-0079.

Meyer, M. C., Johnston, A. M., Crocker, A. M., & Heil, S. H. (2015). Methadone and buprenorphine for opioid dependence during pregnancy: A retrospective cohort study. *Journal of Addiction Medicine, 9*(2), 81–86. https://doi.org/10.1097/adm.0000000000000092.

Moore, E. R., Anderson, G. C., Bergman, N., & Dowswell, T. (2012). Early skin-to-skin contact for mothers and their healthy newborn infants. *Cochrane Database of Systematic Reviews, 5*, CD003519. https://doi.org/10.1002/14651858.CD003519.pub3.

National institute for Children's Health Quality. (2020). *A mother-centered approach to treating neonatal abstinence syndrome*. Retrieved from https://www.nichq.org/insight/mother-centered-approach-treating-neonatal-abstinence-syndrome#

Newman, A., Davies, G. A., Dow, K., Holmes, B., Macdonald, J., Mcknight, S., & Newton, L. (2015). Rooming-in care for infants of opioid-dependent mothers: Implementation and evaluation at a tertiary care hospital. *Canadian Family Physician, 61*, 555–561.

O'Connor, A., Vietze, P. M., Sherrod, K. B., Sandler, H. M., & Altemeirer, W. A. (1980). Reduced incidence of parenting inadequacy following rooming-in. *Pediatrics, 66*(2), 176–182.

O'Grady, M. J., Hopewell, J., & White, M. J. (2009). Management of neonatal abstinence syndrome: A national survey and review of practice. *Archives of Disease in Childhood-Fetal and Neonatal Edition, 94*(4), F249–F252. https://doi.org/10.1136/adc.2008.152769.

Oei, J. L. (2019). After NAS. *Seminars in Fetal and Neonatal Medicine, 24*, 161–165. https://doi.org/10.1016/j.siny.2019.01.012.

Paltrow, L. M., & Flavin, J. (2013). Arrests of and forced interventions on pregnant women in the United States, 1973–2005: Implications for women's legal status and public health. *Journal of Health Politics, Policy and Law, 38*(2), 299–343.

Patrick, S. W. (2015). The triple aim for neonatal abstinence syndrome. *The Journal of Pediatrics, 167*(6), 1189–1191. https://doi.org/10.1016/j.jpeds.2015.09.047.

Patrick, S. W., Schumacher, R. E., Benneyworth, B. D., Krans, E. E., McAllister, J. M., & Davis, M. M. (2012). Neonatal abstinence syndrome and associated health care expenditures: United States, 2000–2009. *JAMA, 307*(18), 1934–1940. https://doi.org/10.1001/jama.2012.3951.

Patrick, S. W., Davis, M. M., Lehmann, C. U., & Cooper, W. O. (2015). Increasing incidence and geographic distribution of neonatal abstinence syndrome: United States 2009 to 2012. *Journal of Perinatology, 35*(8), 650–655. https://doi.org/10.1038/jp.2015.36.

Patrick, S. W., Schumacher, R. E., Horbar, J. D., Buus-Frank, M. E., Edwards, E. M., Morrow, K. A., Ferrelli, K. R., Picarillo, A. P., Gupta, M., & Soll, R. F. (2016). Improving care for neonatal abstinence syndrome. *Pediatrics, 137*(5), 1–8. https://doi.org/10.1542/peds.2015-3835.

Patrick, S. W., Faherty, L. J., Dick, A. W., Scott, T. A., Dudley, J., & Stein, B. D. (2019). Association among county-level economic factors, clinician supply, metropolitan or rural location, and neonatal abstinence syndrome. *JAMA, 321*(4), 385–393. https://doi.org/10.1001/jama.2018.20851.

Porowski, A. W., Burgdorf, K., & Herrell, J. M. (2004). Effectiveness and sustainability of residential substance abuse treatment programs for pregnant and parenting women. *Evaluation and Program Planning, 27*(2), 191–198. https://doi.org/10.1016/j.evalprogplan.2004.01.008.

Pritham, U. A. (2013). Breastfeeding promotion for management of neonatal abstinence syndrome. *Journal of Obstetric, Gynecologic, & Neonatal Nursing, 42*(5), 517–526. https://doi.org/10.1111/1552-6909.12242

Prodromidis, M., Field, T., Arendt, R., Singer, L., Yando, R., & Bendell, D. (1995). Mothers touching newborns: A comparison of rooming-in versus minimal contact. *Birth, 22*, 196–200. https://doi.org/10.1111/j.1523-536X.1995.tb00258.x.

Raeside, L. (2003). Attitudes of staff towards mothers affected by substance abuse. *British Journal of Nursing, 12*, 302–310. https://doi.org/10.12968/bjon.2003.12.5.11176.

Sarkar, S., & Donn, S. M. (2006). Management of neonatal abstinence syndrome in neonatal intensive care units: A national survey. *Journal of Perinatology, 26*(1), 15–17. https://doi.org/10.1038/sj.jp.7211427.

Schiff, D. M., Nielsen, T., Terplan, M., Hood, M., Bernson, D., Diop, H., Bharel, M., Wilens, T. E., LaRochelle, M., Walley, A. Y., & Land, T. (2018). Fatal and nonfatal overdose among pregnant and postpartum women in Massachusetts. *Obstetrics and Gynecology, 132*(2), 466–474. https://doi.org/10.1097/AOG.0000000000002734.

Sebastiani, G., Borrás-Novell, C., Casanova, M. A., Pascual Tutusaus, M., Ferrero Martínez, S., Gómez Roig, M. D., & García-Algar, O. (2018). The effects of alcohol and drugs of abuse on maternal nutritional profile during pregnancy. *Nutrients, 10*(8), 1008. https://doi.org/10.3390/nu10081008.

Stein, M. D., Conti, M. T., Kenney, S., Anderson, B. J., Flori, J. N., Risi, M. M., & Bailey, G. L. (2017). Adverse childhood experience effects on opioid use initiation, injection drug use, and overdose among persons with opioid use disorder. *Drug and Alcohol Dependence, 179*, 325–329. https://doi.org/10.1016/j.drugalcdep.2017.07.007

Stone, R. (2015). Pregnant women and substance use: Fear, stigma, and barriers to care. *Health and Justice, 3*(1), 1–15. https://doi.org/10.1186/s40352-015-0015-5.

Strahan, A. E., Guy, G. P., Bohm, M., Frey, M., & Ko, J. Y. (2020). Neonatal abstinence syndrome incidence and health care costs in the United States, 2016. *JAMA Pediatrics, 174*(2), 200–202. https://doi.org/10.1001/jamapediatrics.2019.4791.

Substance Abuse and Mental Health Services Administration (SAMHSA). (2015). *Substance abuse and mental health services administration federal guidelines for opioid treatment programs* (HHS Publication No. (SMA) PEP15-FEDGUIDEOTP). Rockville: Substance Abuse and Mental Health Services Administration. Retrieved from https://store.samhsa.gov/product/Federal-Guidelines-for-Opioid-Treatment-Programs/PEP15-FEDGUIDEOTP

Substance Abuse and Mental Health Services Administration (SAMHSA). (2016). *A collaborative approach to the treatment of pregnant women with opioid use disorders* (HHS Publication No. (SMA) 16-4978). Rockville: Substance Abuse and Mental Health Services Administration. Retrieved from https://store.samhsa.gov/product/A--Collaborative-Approach-to-the-Treatment-of-Pregnant-Women-with-Opioid-Use-Disorders/SMA16-4978

Substance Abuse and Mental Health Services Administration (SAMHSA). (2018). *Clinical guidance for treating pregnant and parenting women with opioid use disorder and their infants* (HHS Publication No. (SMA) 18-5054). Rockville: Substance Abuse and Mental Health Services Administration. Retrieved from https://store.samhsa.gov/shin/content//SMA18-5054c/SMA18-5054.pdf

U.S. Department of Health and Human Services, Health Resources and Services Administration (HRSA), (2018). *HRSA's home visiting program: Supporting families impacted by opioid use and neonatal abstinence syndrome*. Rockville: U.S. Department of Health and Human Services. Retrieved from https://mchb.hrsa.gov/sites/default/files/mchb/MaternalChildHealthInitiatives/HomeVisiting/MIECHV-Opioid-NAS-Resource.pdf

Villegas, N. A., Chodhury, S. M., Mitrani, V. B., & Guerra, J. (2016). Mothers in substance abuse recovery: Perspectives on motivators, challenges, and family involvement. *International Journal of High Risk Behaviors and Addiction, 6*(1), e32558. https://doi.org/10.5812/ijhrba.32558.

Vogel, L. (2018). Newborns exposed to opioids need mothers more than NICU, say pediatricians. *Canadian Medical Association Journal, 190*(4), E123. https://doi.org/10.1503/cmaj.109-5550.

Winkelman, T. N., Villapiano, N., Kozhimannil, K. B., Davis, M. M., & Patrick, S. W. (2018). Incidence and costs of neonatal abstinence syndrome among infants with Medicaid: 2004–2014. *Pediatrics, 141*(4), e20173520. https://doi.org/10.1542/peds.2017-3520.

Wu, D., & Carre, C. (2018). The impact of breastfeeding on health outcomes for infants diagnosed with neonatal abstinence syndrome: A review. *Cureus, 10*(7). https://doi.org/10.7759/cureus.3061.

Chapter 5
Adverse Childhood Experiences and Addiction

Jennifer Hays-Grudo, Amanda Sheffield Morris, Erin L. Ratliff, and Julie M. Croff

Two decades of research on adverse childhood experiences (ACEs) and a half century of research on child abuse and neglect provide evidence that early life mistreatment and family dysfunction increase the risk of subsequent use and abuse of mood-altering substances. In the original ACEs study of more than 17,000 patients, most of whom were middle-class, middle-aged, and non-Hispanic Caucasian, having four or more of the 10 identified ACEs (mental, physical, sexual abuse; mental, physical neglect; parental substance use, criminality, mental illness, divorce; domestic violence) increased the risk of self-reported alcoholism seven-fold, of illicit drug use 4.5-fold, and of injected drug use 11-fold (Anda et al. 2006; Dube et al. 2001, 2003). Similar findings have been documented in other large population samples in the United States and Europe, with drug and alcohol abuse increasing with number of ACEs in a dose-response effect (Campbell et al. 2016; Merrick et al. 2018).

The relationship between ACEs and substance abuse is even more pronounced in adolescents and young adults living in lower-income and higher-crime neighborhoods than the original ACEs study population (Allem et al. 2015; Mersky et al.

Preparation of this chapter was supported by a Centers of Biomedical Research Excellence grant (P20GM199097, PD: Jennifer Hays-Grudo; National Institutes of Health) and 3/6 Planning for the HEALthy Early Development Study (R34DA050237; MPIs: Julie M. Croff & Amanda S. Morris).

J. Hays-Grudo (✉)
Oklahoma State University Center for Health Sciences, Tulsa, OK, USA
e-mail: jennifer.hays.grudo@okstate.edu

A. S. Morris · E. L. Ratliff
Oklahoma State University, Tulsa, OK, USA
e-mail: amanda.morris@okstate.edu; erin.ratliff@okstate.edu

J. M. Croff
National Center for Wellness and Recovery, Oklahoma State University Center for Health Sciences, Tulsa, OK, USA
e-mail: julie.croff@okstate.edu

J. M. Croff, J. Beaman (eds.), *Family Resilience and Recovery from Opioids and Other Addictions*, Emerging Issues in Family and Individual Resilience,
https://doi.org/10.1007/978-3-030-56958-7_5

2013; Wade et al. 2014). Among these adolescents and young adults, ACEs predict binge drinking after controlling for parent alcoholism (Shin et al. 2009), age of drinking onset (Rothman et al. 2008), and adult alcohol problem drinking (Strine et al. 2012; Loudermilk et al. 2018). ACEs have been found to predict problem alcohol use among young men entering the Marine Corps (Young et al. 2006) and alcohol misuse and alcohol-related risky behaviors in US soldiers returning from war zones, even after adjusting for mental illness and combat exposure.

Current theories on ACEs and addiction acknowledge that early life adversity dysregulates biological and behavioral responses to stress and negative emotions, increasing the likelihood of exogenous substance use for mood regulation; thereby increasing the risk of psychological addiction and physical dependence. Attempts to regulate negative affective states create an additional burden, as the addiction is an adverse experience for children in the household, perpetuating cycles of childhood adversity. This chapter focuses on the points at which ACEs intersect with development and family functioning in ways that can lead to substance use and abuse as well as interventions, policies, and programs that can help adult family members recover from the effects of ACEs to prevent the cycle of adversity and addiction in subsequent generations.

1 Enduring Effects of Adverse Childhood Experiences (ACEs)

The powerful and enduring effects of ACEs have been explained using a number of paradigms and theoretical perspectives. Each of the major approaches is summarized in this section in order to provide a framework for understanding the multiple systems affected by early life stress and suggest effective targets for intervention in the context of substance use disorders.

One of the first approaches to understanding the effects of early life adversity on biobehavioral functioning focused on the effects of stress on developing systems (McEwen 1998). *Allostasis* refers to the body's attempt to maintain equilibrium in response to stressful events, i.e., regaining stability through change (Sterling and Eyer 1988). Allostasis refers to the body's ability to appropriately adapt to stressful stimuli by eliciting and coordinating responses from multiple systems including the nervous, cardiovascular, metabolic, and immune systems. This physiological regulation operates through the body's neuroendocrine stress response system – the hypothalamic-pituitary-adrenal (HPA) axis (Heim et al. 2008; Ramsay and Woods 2014). Stressors activate the hypothalamus to signal the pituitary, which then signals the adrenal gland where adrenaline and cortisol are released. Adrenaline acts to increase heart rate, blood pressure, and the production of glucose and fats. Cortisol, a stress hormone, acts to prepare the body for what is colloquially referred to as the *fight, flight, or freeze* response by inhibiting insulin and flooding the body with glucose. Though this response is adaptive in short-term emergency situations, chronic activation of the HPA axis can have detrimental effects on the brain and body (Heim et al. 2008; McEwen 2003). For example, Heim et al. (2008) found childhood trauma was associated with a sensitization of the HPA axis stress response as well as an increased risk for depression in adulthood. Termed *allostatic load* by McEwen (1998), this persistent wear and tear on the brain and body resulting from experiences of adversity during childhood can become biologically embedded, altering developmental states and dysregulating normal stress responses (Hertzman 2012). Moreover, human and animal research indicates that the biological embedding of stress is associated with changes in brain structure and function (Nelson 2013; Pechtel and Pizzagalli 2011; Teicher and Samson 2016).

1.1 Effects of ACEs on Neurodevelopment

ACES have a profound impact on the developing brain, altering both brain structure and function (Teicher and Samson 2016; Thomason and Marusak 2017). Neuroimaging studies have found decreased hippocampal volume in adults with a history of child maltreatment (Geuze et al. 2005; Teicher and Samson 2016). As part of the limbic system, the hippocampus plays a significant role in memory, learning, and emotions. Furthermore, the hippocampus has been found to regulate activation of the hypothalamus in response to stressors and, therefore, have direct influence on HPA axis responsivity to stressor. Early life adversity can lead to damage to the hippocampus resulting in an altered stress response (Riem et al. 2015). Hippocampal volume is correlated with memory retrieval and cognitive abilities. Therefore, ACES and academic performance, and later economic earnings, could be linked through the effect of adversity on the hippocampus (Frodl et al. 2006).

The amygdala, also found within the limibic system, is also affected by early experiences of adversity, although findings differ by age. Maltreated young children have increased amygdala volume, whereas adolescents and adults with histories of childhood maltreatment have decreased amygdala volume (Fareri and Tottenham 2016; Teicher and Samson 2016). The amygdala plays a significant role in the processing of emotional stimuli; thus, it may be that an enlargement occurs in early childhood, but sensitization to stressors leads to a decrease in volume throughout adolescence and adulthood (Teicher et al. 2016). Studies of amygdala function consistently find increased amygdala responsivity to emotional stimuli in children, adolescents, and adults who have experienced early life adversity and maltreatment (Fareri and Tottenham 2016; Swartz et al. 2015; Teicher and Samson 2016). This heightened reactivity in the amygdala may increase psychological vulnerability through alteration of the stress response.

1.2 Effects of ACES on Executive Function and Regulation

In addition to the hippocampus and amygdala, structural and functional changes have been found in the prefrontal cortex of individuals with a history of childhood maltreatment (Teicher and Samson 2016; Van der Kolk 2003). The prefrontal cortex is responsible for higher-order cognitive function including decision-making, self-referential processing, and emotion awareness and regulation. Development of the prefrontal cortex is protracted across childhood and adolescence (Cook et al. 2017). Research with children and adolescents who have experienced childhood maltreatment shows delayed development of the prefrontal cortex, resulting in difficulties in decision-making, abstract reasoning, and behavioral inhibition (Cook et al. 2017; Van der Kolk 2003). This impaired functioning in the prefrontal cortex may be particularly detrimental during late adolescence when social and cognitive demands increase (Van der Kolk 2003). Studies of adults yield similar patterns of results from childhood adversity on PFC form and function. Van Harmelen et al. (2010, 2014) found reduced medial prefrontal cortex volume in adults with a history of childhood emotional maltreatment as well as reduced activation in the medial prefrontal cortex during a cognitive task but hyperactivation of the amygdala during an emotion processing task. The inferior frontal gyrus is a region within the prefrontal cortex important for impulse control and emotion regulation—possibly another mechanism underlying ACES and risky behavior (Barch et al. 2018; Luby et al. 2017). In a longitudinal study examining ACES and brain function, researchers found higher ACE scores were related to reduced inferior frontal gyrus (IFG) volume, with altered IFG connectivity related to later externalizing issues. Taken together, these findings lend support to the idea that ACES can disrupt neurodevelopment resulting in impaired social, cognitive, and emotional development. When individuals are unable to regulate behavioral and emotional expressions, they may adopt avoidant and maladaptive coping habits such as substance abuse.

1.3 Effects of ACEs on Parent–Child Attachment and Interpersonal Relationships

Unlike natural disasters, pandemics, poverty, war, mass migration, and other adversities that expose children to trauma, the family dysfunction, abuse, and neglect referenced in the ACEs survey involve an element of betrayal. Children who have experienced abuse or neglect are less likely to develop secure attachment styles (Riggs and Kaminski 2010), typically adopting either anxious or avoidant patterns of relating to others. The effect of childhood trauma on adult anxious and avoidant attachment styles has been found to be mediated by emotion dysregulation (Espeleta et al. 2017) and patterns of processing sensory information which are linked to specific brain regions and networks (Crittenden and Landini 2011). Many studies document the effects of early life trauma and insecure attachment to long-term problems with forming close and supportive social bonds with others (Caldwell et al. 2011) and with forming secure attachments with one's own babies and children (Ainsworth 1973). A recent meta-analysis of 34 studies investigating the relationship between attachment and substance use found that insecure attachment is a significant vulnerability factor for the development of addiction (Fairbairn et al. 2018). Conversely, the functional, behavioral, and social impairments associated with substance use disorders may also hinder the formation of secure attachment between parents and very young children.

Strathearn and colleagues have identified three neurobiological pathways by which insecure attachment and adverse childhood experiences increase susceptibility to substance abuse and addiction (Strathearn et al. 2019). Examining both animal and human studies linking ACEs to addiction, they propose a model in which modifications at the molecular, neuroendocrinal, and behavioral levels in three systems—dopamine (reward/habit formation), oxytocin (affiliation), and glucocorticoid (stress response)—result in increased likelihood of substance use, increased susceptibility to addiction, and subsequent impaired parental caregiving and lifelong insecure patterns of attachment. This model may have utility for prevention and intervention programs by identifying unique pathways for different types of substances based on the type of early trauma and insecure attachment patterns. They propose that adverse experiences that alter dopamine receptor expression and production and alter brain reward sensitivity areas (e.g., ventral striatum) increase novelty-seeking, risk-taking behavior, and depression, which may increase susceptibility to stimulants (cocaine, methamphetamines). Adverse experiences that predominately affect the oxytocin (OT) system result in differences in OT receptor expression and OT production; alter sensitivity to social cues in the hypothalamus and prefrontal cortex; increase social isolation, impaired attachments, and emotional pain; and thus increase vulnerability to the effects of opioids. Finally, as described in the previous section, adversities that cause modifications in the glucocorticoid or stress response system modify gene expression and production, altering brain regions sensitive to glucocorticoids (e.g., amygdala, hippocampus), increasing anxiety and susceptibility depressants such as alcohol, cannabis, and benzodiazepines (Strathearn et al. 2019). Considerable evidence from animal models supports the unique effects of different types, severity, and chronicity on each of these systems at the molecular, neuroendocrine, and behavioral levels, and more research with human subjects is warranted. As adversities often co-occur, future interventions may be improved by acknowledging the multiple pathways through which adversity and addictions are transmitted via parenting and attachment styles in mothers with substance abuse disorders.

1.4 *Effects of Biobehavioral Adaptations Associated with ACEs on Addictive Behaviors*

Neurobiological effects of early life trauma also contribute to substance use behaviors through mental health symptomology. Notably, early use of alcohol or marijuana may alleviate symptoms of early life adversity, like depression and anxiety (Chu et al. 2013; Heim and Nemeroff 2001). Early substance use behavior acts to reinforce continued use in two distinct ways: (1) substance use removes the negative stimulus and (2) the intoxication associated with use is a proximal reinforcer for the use behavior. Use of alcohol and marijuana can exacerbate symptoms of anxiety and depression (Bonn-Miller et al. 2007; Roelofs 1985; Laine et al. 1999), thereby driving additional substance use behavior. As biological tolerance increases, individuals may seek out stronger substances to remove the negative stimulus of anxiety. Symptoms associated with early life adversity, therefore, can drive patterns of increased use of alcohol and other substances resulting in dependence.

While alcohol and marijuana are typically the most accessible drugs, the risk of addiction to these drugs from just a few uses is low. More potent dopaminergic releases are experienced from opioids, including heroin, and methamphetamine; making these drugs highly addictive from a single-use. Because the brain is still developing, adolescence and young adulthood remain a critical period of risk for development of substance use disorders. Disruptions in brain development occur across three areas: the basal ganglia, the extended amygdala, and the prefrontal cortex. The basal ganglia are involved in habit formation and reward systems (Kalivas and Volkow 2005). The extended amygdala is involved in stress response and interacts directly with the hypothalamus and pituitary gland, whose role is notable in the *fight or flight* response as noted earlier (Davis et al. 2010). Finally, prefrontal cortex is responsible for executive function, including task prioritization, time management, decision-making, and emotion and impulse regulation (Ball et al. 2011). Notably, the brain systems interrupted by early life adversity are also interrupted and damaged by substance use disorders.

Early life adversity also impacts the ability to recover from a substance use disorder. Early life adversity directly affects the recovery capital of an individual (Cleveland et al. 2020), often resulting in fewer social relationships to support recovery. Social relationships also impact the economic capital accessible to an individual with substance use disorder: treatment is expensive and often needs to be repeated for this chronic, relapsing condition. Notably, early life adversity negatively impacts the ability to engage in treatment by reducing both participation and engagement of psychosocial treatment (Somer 2003). Therefore, individuals with early life adversity may need more economic and social capital to be successful in recovery because it will take them more attempts and more time to engage in treatment.

2 Treating Addiction by Healing the Effects of ACEs

Viewing substance abuse and addiction through the lens of childhood adversity provides an alternative to the disease model, which defines addiction as a "chronic, relapsing disorder characterized by compulsive drug seeking, continued use despite harmful consequences, and long-lasting changes in the brain" (https://www.drugabuse.gov/publications/media-guide/science-drug-use-addiction-basics). Nor does it consider addiction as a moral failure, an example of individuals making poor choices or failing to exert self-control. Rather, early physically or emotionally painful experiences are seen as the primary source of alterations made by exquisitely interconnected biobehavioral systems to reduce stress and increase immediate survival. These short-term adaptive responses may have injurious long-term consequences for physiological systems (immunologic, brain structure, and function) and the developments of executive function skills, such as the ability to set goals, solve problems, manage negative thoughts, control emotional and behavioral responses, and form close and mutually rewarding relationships with others.

As these impairments increase susceptibility to substance use, they also provide targets for interventions to remove underlying vulnerabilities to addiction. We focus on three types of interventions that address deficits that increase risk for addition: mindfulness and other body-based programs to repair dysfunctional stress response systems; enriched environment programs (e.g., PACEs) to support the development of executive function skills in adults and children, and attachment-promoting therapy for parents and children (e.g., ABC) to reduce intergenerational transmission of adversity and addiction. Hays-Grudo and Morris (2020) have suggested that it may be useful to view the original ACEs pyramid (Felitti et al. 1998) as an ACEs iceberg. When viewed as an iceberg, the consequences of ACEs that are unseen or below the surface, i.e., altered neurodevelopment and attending social, cognitive, and emotional deficits, provide better targets for prevention and early intervention efforts than the more visible problem behaviors or chronic condition. Thus, the next section will describe interventions that address the underlying causes of observable health-harming behaviors such as the substance use, the disease process, and the conditions resulting from addiction.

2.1 *Mindfulness-Based Interventions*

One of the most well-researched interventions to improve the body's ability to regulate stress and negative emotions is Mindfulness-Based Stress Reduction (MBSR; Kabat-Zinn 2005). MBSR was originally developed to reduce stress and improve health and well-being by Dr. Jon Kabat-Zinn at the University of Massachusetts and has been used to improve outcomes for patients suffering from a variety of chronic ailments as well as healthy individuals seeking skills to cope with the stresses of daily life. A typical training course consists of weekly 2- to 3-h sessions for 8 weeks plus one all-day session, group meditation and yoga practice, and homework assignments to apply mindfulness to everyday activities (e.g., walking and eating). MBSR practice focuses on experiencing objective and sustained awareness of physical sensations, perceptions, thoughts, and feelings with no corresponding judgment. Mindfulness-based programs may be useful in reducing substance abuse as they appear to develop new neural connections related to impairments in executive function and reduce the process of craving and suffering in addiction treatment. Research documents improvement in such executive function skills as focused attention, emotion regulation, emotion processing, and self-awareness, with corresponding changes in associated brain regions (Gotink et al. 2016; Hatchard et al. 2017; Tang et al. 2015). Research also indicates that MBSR and adapted mindfulness programs are effective for reducing emotional pain and craving associated with substance use and addiction (Black 2014). In a randomized clinical trial, mindfulness-based relapse prevention programs was more effective than cognitive behavioral relapse prevention or treatment as usual in prevention relapse to heavy drug or alcohol use one year after treatment (Bowen et al. 2014).

2.2 *Protective and Compensatory Experiences (PACEs) for Children and Adults*

For more than six decades, researchers have studied the characteristics of children, families, and communities which promote resilience (Rutter 1987), defined by Masten as "the capacity of a dynamic system to adapt successfully to disturbances that threaten system function, viability, or development" (Masten 2014, p. 6). Luthar et al. (2000) note that two elements are required for resilience to occur: exposure to threat or severe adversity and positive adaptation despite significant attacks on development. From this body of knowledge, (Morris and Hays-Grudo 2014; Morris et al. 2018) identified 10 environmental characteristics that appear to buffer children from the effects of parental substance abuse and other ACEs and may be helpful to adults working to overcome the effects of their own adverse childhoods and subsequent substance use. These Protective and Compensatory Experiences (PACEs) can be compared to consist of five types of relationship patterns and five categories of resources that promote positive adaptation and development in children exposed to significant adversity. Research indicates that both relationships and resources are necessary to provide the nurture, stability, and environmental assets needed for healthy child outcomes (Duncan and Brooks-Gunn 2000; McLoyd 1998; Shonkoff 2010). These experiences provide the context for the development of biobehavioral regulation of stress, emotion regulation, and social attachments even when family dysfunction and parental impairment jeopardize healthy development (Hays-Grudo and Morris 2020; Morris et al. 2018).

Relationships that serve as PACEs include (a) unconditional love from a parent or other primary caregiver; (b) having a best friend; (c) volunteering or helping others in the community; (d) being part of a social group; and (e) having a mentor or supportive adult outside the family. The resources we identified as PACEs include (f) living in a clean, uncluttered home with adequate food; (g) having opportunities to learn (access to good schools); (h) having an engaging hobby, creative or intellectual pursuit; (i) being physically active either in leisure activities or in organized sports; (j) having regular routines and consistent, fair rules to follow. It should be noted that many of these experiences are less accessible to children growing up in low-income households and neighborhoods. This is an issue that is often neglected in policy discussions about whether children have access to after-school activities in rural communities, in single-parent households, and in low-income neighborhoods. The very children who may be most at risk due to poverty and its associated stressors also have the least access to the resources and experiences that would help buffer their negative effects. The importance of PACEs in the context of parental or family addiction is the importance of communities, extended family and friends, teachers, and other caring adults identifying opportunities to provide supportive relationships and resources for children at risk.

The importance of relationships and resources for adults struggling to overcome a history of trauma is less well researched but may be helpful in the context of recovery and relearning life skills and behavior patterns that prevent relapse. Substance-abusing adults who grew up in dysfunctional homes may gain much-needed therapy and treatment during the course of their journey from addiction to sobriety, but little attention is given to learning how highly functioning families prioritize and organize their time and material resources. Adults who create a PACEs plan for themselves and their families are beginning the process of establishing and maintaining these priorities, creating environments with the support and routines that maintain physical, social, and emotional health (Hays-Grudo and Morris 2020). Parents who have struggled with substance abuse can help mitigate the effects of that and other related ACEs in their children's lives by increasing their exposure to these protective and compensatory experiences (Breakout Box 5.1).

Breakout Box 5.1. Focus on Practice

While working as a service provider in the community, I often would learn about my client's early childhood experience in several different ways. Sometimes, I learned about this information from the clinical record. Other times, I would gather the information from family reports. I also learned about a client's early childhood experiences during conversations with them. Through my experiences, I found that most clients were willing to provide this information, especially if I gently approach the subject. However, from time to time, I would have a client that wouldn't want to disclose this information. Sharing this information is critical as these childhood experiences need to be addressed, though it may depends on the client and their current situation. Among adults who experienced negative events when young, I would say that one common theme among resilient adults is having at least one positive relationship with an adult during their childhood, especially an adult who was willing to be there for them. With my clients, if these early experiences are causing problems – such as difficulty forming positive interpersonal relationships or ongoing depression – I often encourage them to seek out professional help. For individuals who serve as service providers in the community, my number one recommendation is to get training on becoming trauma aware, such as being able to identify different traumatic experiences people may have experienced during their childhood or even more recently. This type of training needs to be ongoing and refreshed on a regular basis. In addition to service providers, community leaders can help individuals who experience traumatic events by first supporting programs the give children access to positive experiences outside of the home. As far as helping adults who experienced traumatic events as children, supporting community mental health services is a great place to start.

-Kris Stallard, Community Service Navigator

2.3 Attachment-Based Intervention to Interrupt Intergenerational Patterns

When parents have had many ACEs themselves, it may be difficult for them to provide sensitive, nurturing care to their children. Such parents often did not experience sensitive, nurturing care, and in fact, may have experienced harsh or frightening behaviors. These prior experiences make it difficult for parents to "provide to their children what they didn't get" (Sroufe, personal communication, June 5, 1995). However, the children of parents who have had many ACEs especially need responsive caregiving. Nurturing care is especially important for young children who have experienced early adversity. For example, we have found that young foster children developed disorganized attachments at high rates if their foster parents were not nurturing (Dozier et al. 2001). Young children who have experienced adversity are also at risk for physiological and behavioral dysregulation (Bernard et al. 2010). They need parents who are well attuned to their signals who can help them develop adequate self-regulation. In addition, when parents behave in frightening ways, it undermines children's ability to form secure attachments and to develop adequate regulatory capabilities (Main and Hesse 1990). These difficulties are exacerbated when parents have substance abuse disorders (Kim et al. 2017). Therefore, even if parents have improved in their ability to be nurturing to their distressed child and to be highly attuned to children's signals, the gains will not be realized in children's outcomes if parents are frightening.

Attachment and Biobehavioral Catch-up (ABC) was designed to improve these three identified goals in parents who had ACEs and other high-risk parents. Specifically, they help to nurture their distressed child, follow their child's lead (i.e., demonstrate to child that they are well attuned to signals), and avoid frightening behavior. ABC is implemented through 10 sessions conducted in parents' homes, with children, parents, and others in the home invited to join. The sessions include frequent feedback to parents regarding how their own behaviors are illustrative of nurturance and following the lead. This feedback provides parents practice in the targeted behaviors and has been shown to enhance parental sensitivity (Caron et al. 2018).

The efficacy of the ABC intervention has been assessed through randomized clinical trials. Relative to parents in the control intervention, parents assigned to the ABC intervention were more sensitive to their children and less intrusive immediately after the intervention and three years later (Bick and Dozier 2013). Children whose parents received ABC showed secure, organized attachments more than children whose parents received the control intervention (Bernard et al. 2012) and better regulation of behavior and physiology (e.g., Bernard et al. 2015; Bick et al. 2019; Tabachnick et al. 2019) than children whose parents received the control condition, with those changes sustained at least 8 years following the intervention.

3 Implications

3.1 Implications for Understanding Family Resilience

Many of the PACEs mentioned previously include factors that promote family resilience. For example, nurturing relationships and unconditional love support cohesiveness in families, and structure, rituals, and routine are all facets of families that can foster resilience and adaptability. Indeed, family systems may be characterized as adaptive or maladaptive (see Henry et al. 2015), and characteristics of families can serve as protective factors against substance use disorders or can exacerbate risk. Developmentally, families can adapt to stressors caused by addiction and can provide great support during treatment and recovery. Among mothers, having a young child can act as a protective factor against substance use and a strong driver for successful treatment. Programs such as ABC likely help to rewire reward systems so that positive interactions with young children are praised, increasing their likelihood in the future. During adolescence, families can protect children from addiction through rules, support, and involvement and by modeling appropriate behavior with legal substance use. In general, the family plays a major role in creating an environment that leads to addiction through ACEs and other maladaptive patterns or can promote resilience and healing from addiction in individuals and youth.

3.2 Implications for Practice and Policy

The research reviewed in this chapter highlights the relationship between substance abuse and the family. Children who grow up in homes with substance-abusing parents are at risk for other forms of adversity, all of which impair the development of healthy cognitive, social, and emotional functioning. This places them at increased risk of early exposure to substances, increases the susceptibility to addiction, and reduces the internal and external resources with which to overcome both adversity and addiction. Just as the family can be one of the primary risk factors for addiction, the family can also be a powerful source of resilience for children. We have identified 10 PACEs that parents can implement in their families to promote resilience for themselves, their children, and their family as a whole. Interventions that increase parents' responsiveness to their young children, such as the Attachment and Biobehavioral Catch-up, have demonstrated enduring changes in vulnerable children and their parents' biological stress responses and attachment security because the program builds on the strong desire of parents and children to have secure attachments. Intergenerational patterns of adversity and addictions can be interrupted. By 2017, more than 2.2 million children in the United States had been exposed to childhood adversity because of the opioid epidemic (UHF 2019), which drove up rates of substance use disorders to highly addictive substances. Substance abuse treatment is enhanced by incorporating programs that address these intergenerational patterns and provide opportunities to create more supportive and resourceful environments in which to recover from adversity.

4 Conclusions and Future Directions

Childhood adversity is significant predictor of mental illness and substance abuse disorders, as early life stress alters both biological and behavioral adaptations to stress, decreasing the individual's ability and capacity to manage negative emotions and increasing the likelihood of dependence on mood-altering substances (Kirsch et al. 2020). There is sufficient evidence that programs and policies that promote positive parenting and family functioning can buffer the effects of early adversity. Interventions that promote secure attachment, such as Attachment Biobehavioral Catch-up (ABC), show promise for interrupting the intergenerational cycle of adversity and addiction. Policies and programs that ensure access to Protective and Compensatory Experiences (PACEs) within families and communities also show promise for protecting children who are exposed to ACEs and family addiction.

The current epidemic of substance abuse disorders and the effects of addiction on children and families warrant changes in both research and practice patterns. One suggestion for future research is the development of improved screening and assessment measures and processes to identify children and adolescents at risk for substance-related vulnerability. The ACEs questionnaire was originally developed for epidemiological research with large populations and may not provide the most sensitive or predictive tool for individual screening or assessment (Anda et al. 2020). New measures could be more sensitive to the types of ACEs that are prevalent, the ACEs that cluster together, the chronicity and severity of the adversity, the age of exposure, and the existence of adversities not originally included in the CDC questionnaire, such as exposure to discrimination based on race, ethnicity, sexual orientation, religion, or other individual characteristics, early medical trauma, peer bullying, or social exclusion.

More research is also needed to develop and evaluate interventions aimed at disrupting the trajectory of youth at risk for substance abuse based on exposure to the types of adversity described previously. These interventions could draw from research suggesting that both individual and group-based programs are required. For example, individual and group-based mindfulness programs show promise, as they help children and youth, as well as adults, develop the capacity to monitor and regulate stress and negative emotions without relying on external substances. Although examples are few, there is emerging evidence that community-wide interventions can be effective in reducing teen substance abuse (Young 2017). In Iceland, the widespread rates of alcohol and other substance abuse in teens led to a committed effort to change as a society, reducing advertising and access to alcohol and instituting adolescent nighttime curfews, but also increasing access to after-school activities and job training programs. Parents were asked to be involved, signing pledges to monitor their teens' activities and not purchase alcohol, tobacco, or other drugs for them. A decade later, not only did rates of teen alcohol and drug use plummet but adolescents reported spending more time with their families and enjoying healthier sports and recreational activities. Intervention research that strengthens the relationships and support within families along with the assets and resources of communities is needed to reduce the effects of ACEs and substance use disorders on future generations.

Glossary of Terms

Addiction a brain disease whose visible symptoms are behaviors
Adversity a host of experiences that can cause serious or chronic stress.
Attachment an emotional bond that connects one person to another
Adverse Childhood Experiences (ACEs) ten potentially traumatic events that occur in childhood (verbal abuse, physical abuse, sexual abuse, physical neglect, emotional neglect, witness interpersonal violence, substance abuse in home, separated/divorced parents, family member incarcerated, family member mentally ill or suicidal)
Protective and Compensatory Experiences (PACEs) ten environmental characteristics that appear to buffer children from the effects of parental substance abuse and other ACEs and may be helpful to adults working to overcome the effects of their own adverse childhoods and subsequent substance use

Questions for Thought and Discussion

1. Think about the concept of "adaptation." How can biological and behavioral adaptations to threatening or dangerous experience during childhood have long-term maladaptive consequences? How would the prevention and treatment of substance use disorders be different if it is thought of as short-term adaptations with long-term consequences?
2. Develop a research question based on one of the assertions made in this chapter, (e.g., that mindfulness practice can reduce substance abuse in teens by improving deficits in executive function skills resulting from ACEs) and design an intervention study to examine it. Include in your research design qualitative as well as quantitative measures to assess the effects of the intervention.
3. The authors propose that clinical practitioners and policy makers should consider the importance of providing enriched environments and supportive relationships for at-risk children and their families. Select five of the PACEs that could be made more accessible to families through existing health care systems, social services, educational systems, or philanthropic programs.

4. Write a letter to the editor of your local newspaper that describes in everyday language the link between ACEs and addiction, including the biological and behavioral effects on child development, the evidence-based programs that can interrupt the cycle of adversity and addition, and why the community would benefit from making such programs more available.

References

Ainsworth, M. D. S. (1973). The development of mother-infant attachment. *Review of Child Development Research, 3*, 1–94.

Allem, J. P., Soto, D. W., Baezconde-Garbanati, L., & Unger, J. B. (2015). Adverse childhood experiences and substance use among Hispanic emerging adults in Southern California. *Addictive Behaviors, 50*, 199–204.

Anda, R. F., Felitti, V. J., Bremner, J. D., Walker, J. D., Whitfield, C., Perry, B. D., et al. (2006). The enduring effects of abuse and related adverse experiences in childhood. A convergence of evidence from neurobiology and epidemiology. *European Archives of Psychiatry and Clinical Neuroscience, 256*(3), 174–186. https://doi.org/10.1007/s00406-005-0624-4.

Anda, R. F., Porter, L. E., & Brown, D. W. (2020). Inside the adverse childhood experience score: Strengths, limitations, and misapplications. American Journal of Preventive Medicine, 59(2), 293–295.

Ball, G., Stokes, P. R., Rhodes, R. A., Bose, S. K., Rezek, I., Wink, A.-M., & Turkheimer, F. E. (2011). Executive functions and prefrontal cortex: A matter of persistence? *Frontiers in Systems Neuroscience, 5*(3), 1–13.

Barch, D. M., Belden, A. C., Tillman, R., Whalen, D., & Luby, J. L. (2018). Early childhood adverse experiences, inferior frontal gyrus connectivity, and the trajectory of externalizing psychopathology. *Journal of the American Academy of Child & Adolescent Psychiatry, 57*(3), 183–190.

Bernard, K., Butzin-Dozier, Z., Rittenhouse, J., & Dozier, M. (2010). Cortisol production patterns in young children living with birth parents vs children placed in foster care following involvement of Child Protective Services. *Archives of Pediatrics and Adolescent Medicine, 164*, 438–443.

Bernard, K., Dozier, M., Bick, J., Lewis-Morrarty, E., Lindhiem, O., & Carlson, E. (2012). Enhancing attachment organization among maltreated infants: Results of a randomized clinical trial. *Child Development, 83*, 623–636.

Bernard, K., Hostinar, C. E., & Dozier, M. (2015). Intervention effects on diurnal cortisol rhythms of CPS-referred infants persist into early childhood: Preschool follow-up results of a randomized clinical trial. *JAMA-Pediatrics, 169*, 112–119.

Bick, J., & Dozier, M. (2013). The effectiveness of an attachment-based intervention in promoting foster mothers' sensitivity toward foster infants. *Infant Mental Health Journal, 34*, 95–103.

Bick, J., Palmwood, E., Zajac, L., Simons, R. F., & Dozier, M. (2019). Early prevention and adverse environments affect neural functioning in middle childhood. *Biological Psychiatry, 85*, 326–335.

Black, D. S. (2014). Mindfulness-based interventions: An antidote to suffering in the context of substance use, misuse, and addiction. *Substance Use & Misuse, 49*(5), 487–491.

Bonn-Miller, M. O., Zvolensky, M. J., Marshall, E. C., & Bernstein, A. (2007). Incremental validity of anxiety sensitivity in relation to marijuana withdrawal symptoms. *Addictive Behaviors, 32*(9), 1843–1851.

Bowen, S., Witkiewitz, K., Clifasefi, S. L., Grow, J., Chawla, N., Hsu, S. H., et al. (2014). Relative efficacy of mindfulness-based relapse prevention, standard relapse prevention, and treatment as usual for substance use disorders: A randomized clinical trial. *JAMA Psychiatry, 71*(5), 547–556.

Blaze, J., & Roth, T. L. (2015, July). Evidence from clinical and animal model studies of the long-term and transgenerational impact of stress on DNA methylation. In Seminars in cell & developmental biology (Vol. 43, pp. 76–84). Academic Press.

Caldwell, J. G., Shaver, P. R., Li, C.-S., & Minzenberg, M. J. (2011). Childhood maltreatment, adult attachment, and depression as predictors of parental self-efficacy in at-risk mothers. *Journal of Aggression, Maltreatment & Trauma, 20*(6), 595–616. https://doi.org/10.1080/10926771.2011.595763.

Campbell, J. A., Walker, R. J., & Egede, L. E. (2016). Associations between adverse childhood experiences, high-risk behaviors, and morbidity in adulthood. *American Journal of Preventative Medicine, 50*(3), 344–352. https://doi.org/10.1016/j.amepre.2015.07.022.

Caron, E., Bernard, K., & Dozier, M. (2018). In-vivo feedback predicts behavioral change in the attachment and biobehavioral catch-up intervention. *Journal of Clinical Child and Adolescent Psychology, 47*, S35–S46.

Chu, D. A., Williams, L. M., Harris, A. W., Bryant, R. A., & Gatt, J. M. (2013). Early life trauma predicts self-reported levels of depressive and anxiety symptoms in nonclinical community adults: Relative contributions of early life stressor types and adult trauma exposure. *Journal of Psychiatric Research, 47*(1), 23–32.

Cleveland, H., Brick, T., Knapp, K., & Croff, J. (2020). Recovery & recovery capital: Aligning measurement with theory and practice. In J. Croff & J. Beaman (Eds.), *Family resilience and recovery: Opioids and other addictions*. Springer. Manuscript submitted for publication.

Cook, A., Spinazzola, J., Ford, J., Lanktree, C., Blaustein, M., Cloitre, M., et al. (2017). Complex trauma in children and adolescents. *Psychiatric Annals, 35*(5), 390–398.

Crittenden, P. M., & Landini, A. (2011). *Assessing adult attachment: A dynamic-maturational approach to discourse analysis*. New York/London: WW Norton & Company.

Davis, M., Walker, D. L., Miles, L., & Grillon, C. (2010). Phasic vs sustained fear in rats and humans: Role of the extended amygdala in fear vs anxiety. *Neuropsychopharmacology, 35*(1), 105–135.

Dozier, M., Stovall, K. C., Albus, K. E., & Bates, B. (2001). Attachment for infants in foster care: The role of caregiver state of mind. *Child Development, 72*, 1467–1477.

Dube, S. R., Anda, R. F., Felitti, V. J., Croft, J. B., Edwards, V. J., & Giles, W. H. (2001). Growing up with parental alcohol abuse: Exposure to childhood abuse, neglect, and household dysfunction. *Child Abuse & Neglect, 25*(12), 1627–1640.

Dube, S. R., Felitti, V. J., Dong, M., Chapman, D. P., Giles, W. H., & Anda, R. F. (2003). Childhood abuse, neglect, and household dysfunction and the risk of illicit drug use: The adverse childhood experiences study. *Pediatrics, 111*(3), 564–572.

Duncan, G. J., & Brooks-Gunn, J. (2000). Family poverty, welfare reform, and child development. *Child Development, 71*(1), 188–196.

Espeleta, H. C., Palasciano-Barton, S., & Messman-Moore, T. L. (2017). The impact of child abuse severity on adult attachment anxiety and avoidance in college women: The role of emotion dysregulation. *Journal of Family Violence, 32*, 399–407. https://doi.org/10.1007/s10896-016-9816-0.

Fairbairn, C. E., Briley, D. A., Kang, D., Fraley, R. C., Hankin, B. L., & Ariss, T. (2018). A meta-analysis of longitudinal associations between substance use and interpersonal attachment security. *Psychological Bulletin, 144*(5), 532.

Fareri, D. S., & Tottenham, N. (2016). Effects of early life stress on amygdala and striatal development. *Developmental Cognitive Neuroscience, 19*, 233–247.

Frodl, T., Schaub, A., Banac, S., Charypar, M., Jäger, M., Kümmler, P., et al. (2006). Reduced hippocampal volume correlates with executive dysfunctioning in major depression. *Journal of Psychiatry and Neuroscience, 31*(5), 316.

Felitti, V. J., Anda, R. F., Nordenberg, D., Williamson, D. F., Spitz, A. M., Edwards, V., & Marks, J. S. (1998). Relationship of childhood abuse and household dysfunction to many of the leading causes of death in adults: The Adverse Childhood Experiences (ACE) Study. *American Journal of Preventive Medicine, 14*(4), 245–258.

Geuze, E. E. J. D., Vermetten, E., & Bremner, J. D. (2005). MR-based in vivo hippocampal volumetrics: 2. Findings in neuropsychiatric disorders. *Molecular Psychiatry, 10*(2), 160–184.

Gotink, R. A., Meijboom, R., Vernooij, M. W., Smits, M., & Hunink, M. M. (2016). 8-week mindfulness based stress reduction induces brain changes similar to traditional long-term meditation practice–a systematic review. *Brain and Cognition, 108*, 32–41.

Hatchard, T., Mioduszewski, O., Zambrana, A., O'Farrell, E., Caluyong, M., Poulin, P. A., & Smith, A. M. (2017). Neural changes associated with mindfulness-based stress reduction (mbsr): Current knowledge, limitations, and future directions. *Psychology & Neuroscience, 10*(1), 41.

Hays-Grudo, J., & Morris, A. S. (2020). *Adverse and protective childhood experiences: A developmental perspective*. Washington, DC: American Psychological Association.

Heim, C., & Nemeroff, C. B. (2001). The role of childhood trauma in the neurobiology of mood and anxiety disorders: Preclinical and clinical studies. *Biological Psychiatry, 49*(12), 1023–1039.

Heim, C., Newport, D. J., Mletzko, T., Miller, A. H., & Nemeroff, C. B. (2008). The link between childhood trauma and depression: Insights from HPA axis studies in humans. *Psychoneuroendocrinology, 33*(6), 693–710.

Henry, C. S., Sheffield Morris, A., & Harrist, A. W. (2015). Family resilience: Moving into the third wave. *Family Relations, 64*(1), 22–43.

Hertzman, C. (2012). Putting the concept of biological embedding in historical perspective. *Proceedings of the National Academy of Sciences*. 201202203.

Kabat-Zinn, J. (2005). *Coming to our senses: Healing ourselves and the world through mindfulness*. New York: Hachette UK.

Kalivas, P. W., & Volkow, N. D. (2005). The neural basis of addiction: A pathology of motivation and choice. *The American Journal of Psychiatry, 162*(8), 1403–1413.

Kim, S., Iyengar, U., Mayes, L. C., Potenza, M. N., Rutherford, H. J., & Strathearn, L. (2017). Mothers with substance addictions show reduced reward responses when viewing their own infant's face. *Human Brain Mapping, 38*(11), 5421–5439.

Kirsch, D., Nemeroff, C. M., & Lippard, E. T. (2020). Early life stress and substance use disorders: Underlying neurobiology and pathways to adverse outcomes. *Adversity and Resilience Science*, 1–19.

Laine, T. P. J., Ahonen, A., Räsänen, P., & Tiihonen, J. (1999). Dopamine transporter availability and depressive symptoms during alcohol withdrawal. *Psychiatry Research: Neuroimaging, 90*(3), 153–157.

Loudermilk, E., Loudermilk, K., Obenauer, J., & Quinn, M. A. (2018). Impact of adverse childhood experiences (ACEs) on adult alcohol consumption behaviors. *Child Abuse & Neglect, 86*, 368–374.

Luby, J. L., Barch, D., Whalen, D., Tillman, R., & Belden, A. (2017). Association between early life adversity and risk for poor emotional and physical health in adolescence: A putative mechanistic neurodevelopmental pathway. *JAMA Pediatrics, 171*(12), 1168–1175.

Luthar, S. S., Cicchetti, D., & Becker, B. (2000). The construct of resilience: A critical evaluation and guidelines for future work. *Child Development, 71*(3), 543–562.

Main, M., & Hesse, E. (1990). Parents' unresolved traumatic experiences are related to infant disorganized attachment status: Is frightened and/or frightening parental behavior the linking mechanism? In M. T. Greenberg, D. Cicchetti, & E. Cummings (Eds.), *Attachment in the preschool years: Theory, research, and intervention* (pp. 161–182). Chicago: University of Chicago Press.

Masten, A. S. (2014). Global perspectives on resilience in children and youth. *Child Development, 85*(1), 6–20.

McEwen, B. S. (1998). Protective and damaging effects of stress mediators. *New England Journal of Medicine, 338*(3), 171–179. https://doi.org/10.1056/NEJM199801153380307.

McEwen, B. S. (2003). Interacting mediators of allostasis and allostatic load: Towards an understanding of resilience in aging. *Metabolism, 52*, 10–16.

McLoyd, V. C. (1998). Socioeconomic disadvantage and child development. *American Psychologist, 53*(2), 185.

Merrick, M. T., Ford, D. C., Ports, K. A., & Guinn, A. S. (2018). Prevalence of adverse childhood experiences from the 2011–2014 behavioral risk factor surveillance system in 23 states. *Journal of the American Medical Association Pediatrics, 172*, 1038–1044.

Mersky, J. P., Topitzes, J., & Reynolds, A. J. (2013). Impacts of adverse childhood experiences on health, mental health, and substance use in early adulthood: A cohort study of an urban, minority sample in the US. *Child Abuse & Neglect, 37*(11), 917–925.

Morris, A. S., Treat, A. E., Hays-Grudo, J., Chesher, T., Williamson, A. C., & Mendez, J. (2018). Integrating research and theory on early relationships to guide intervention and prevention. In A. S. Morris & A. C. Williamson (Eds.), *Building early social and emotional relationships with infants and toddlers* (pp. 1–26). Cham: Springer.

Morris, A. S., & Hays-Grudo, J. (2014). *Protecting parents and children from Adverse Childhood Experiences (ACEs): Preliminary evidence for the validity of the PACEs* (with Amanda Morris). In: Paper presented at the SRCD special topic meeting: New conceptualizations in the study of parenting-at-risk, San Diego.

Nelson, C. A. (2013). Biological embedding of early life adversity. *The Journal of the American Medical Association Pediatrics, 167*(12), 1098–1100.

Pechtel, P., & Pizzagalli, D. A. (2011). Effects of early life stress on cognitive and affective function: An integrated review of human literature. *Psychopharmacology, 214*(1), 55–70.

Riem, M. M., Alink, L. R., Out, D., Van Ijzendoorn, M. H., & Bakermans-Kranenburg, M. J. (2015). Beating the brain about abuse: Empirical and meta-analytic studies of the association between maltreatment and hippocampal volume across childhood and adolescence. *Development and Psychopathology, 27*(2), 507–520.

Riggs, S. A., & Kaminski, P. (2010). Childhood emotional abuse, adult attachment, and depression as predictors of relational adjustment and psychological aggression. *Journal of Aggression, Maltreatment & Trauma, 19*(1), 75–104.

Roelofs, S. M. (1985). Hyperventilation, anxiety, craving for alcohol: A subacute alcohol withdrawal syndrome. *Alcohol, 2*(3), 501–505.

Rothman, E. F., Edwards, E. M., Heeren, T., & Hingson, R. W. (2008). Adverse childhood experiences predict earlier age of drinking onset: Results from a representative US sample of current or former drinkers. *Pediatrics, 122*(2), e298–e304.

Rutter, M. (1987). Psychosocial resilience and protective mechanisms. *American Journal of Orthopsychiatry, 57*(3), 316–331.

Shin, S. H., Edwards, E. M., & Heeren, T. (2009). Child abuse and neglect: Relations to adolescent binge drinking in the national longitudinal study of adolescent health (AddHealth) study. *Addictive Behaviors, 34*(3), 277–280.

Shonkoff, J. P. (2010). Building a new biodevelopmental framework to guide the future of early childhood policy. *Child Development, 81*(1), 357–367.

Somer, E. (2003). Prediction of abstinence from heroin addiction by childhood trauma, dissociation, and extent of psychosocial treatment. *Addiction Research & Theory, 11*(5), 339–348. https://doi.org/10.1080/1606635031000141102.

Strathearn, L., Mertens, C. E., Mayes, L., Rutherford, H., Rajhans, P., Xu, G., Potenza, M. N., & Kim, S. (2019). Pathways relating the neurobiology of attachment to drug addiction. *Frontiers in Psychiatry, 10*, 737.

Strine, T. W., Dube, S. R., Edwards, V. J., Prehn, A. W., Rasmussen, S., Wagenfeld, M., et al. (2012). Associations between adverse childhood experiences, psychological distress, and adult alcohol problems. *American Journal of Health Behavior, 36*(3), 408–423.

Swartz, J. R., Knodt, A. R., Radtke, S. R., & Hariri, A. R. (2015). A neural biomarker of psychological vulnerability to future life stress. *Neuron, 85*(3), 505–511.

Sterling, P., & Eyer, J. (1988). Allostasis; A new paradigm to rxplain srousal pathology. In: S. Fisher, S. & J. Reason, Eds. *Handbook of Life Stress, Cognition and Health* (PP. 629–649). New York: Wiley.

Tabachnick, A., Raby, K. L., Goldstein, A., Zajac, L., & Dozier, M. (2019). Effects of an attachment-based intervention on children's autonomic regulation during middle childhood. *Biological Psychology, 143*, 22–31.

Tang, Y. Y., Holzel, B. K., & Posner, M. I. (2015). The neuroscience of mindfulness meditation. *Nature Reviews Neuroscience, 16*(4), 213–225. https://doi.org/10.1038/nrn3916.

Teicher, M. H., & Samson, J. A. (2016). Annual research review: Enduring neurobiological effects of childhood abuse and neglect. *Journal of Child Psychology and Psychiatry, 57*(3), 241–266. https://doi.org/10.1111/jcpp.12507.

Teicher, M. H., Samson, J. A., Anderson, C. M., & Ohashi, K. (2016). The effects of childhood maltreatment on brain structure, function and connectivity. *Nature Reviews Neuroscience, 17*(10), 652.

Thomason, M. E., & Marusak, H. A. (2017). Toward understanding the impact of trauma on the early developing human brain. *Neuroscience, 342*, 55–67.

United Hospital Fund. (2019). *The ripple effect: Nation and state estimates of the US Opioid epidemics effect on children.*

van Harmelen, A. L., van Tol, M. J., van der Wee, N. J., Veltman, D. J., Aleman, A., Spinhoven, P., et al. (2010). Reduced medial prefrontal cortex volume in adults reporting childhood emotional maltreatment. *Biological Psychiatry, 68*(9), 832–838.

van Harmelen, A. L., van Tol, M. J., Dalgleish, T., van der Wee, N. J., Veltman, D. J., Aleman, A., et al. (2014). Hypoactive medial prefrontal cortex functioning in adults reporting childhood emotional maltreatment. *Social Cognitive and Affective Neuroscience, 9*(12), 2026–2033.

Van der Kolk, B. A. (2003). The neurobiology of childhood trauma and abuse. *Child and Adolescent Psychiatric Clinics, 12*(2), 293–317.

Wade, R., Jr., Shea, J. A., Rubin, D., & Wood, J. (2014). Adverse childhood experiences of low-income urban youth. *Pediatrics, 134*(1), e13–e20. https://doi.org/10.1542/peds.2013-2475.

Young, E. (2017). How Iceland got teens to say no to drugs. *The Atlantic*, 1–15.

Young, S. Y., Hansen, C. J., Gibson, R. L., & Ryan, M. A. (2006). Risky alcohol use, age at onset of drinking, and adverse childhood experiences in young men entering the US Marine Corps. *Archives of Pediatrics & Adolescent Medicine, 160*(12), 1207–1214.

Chapter 6
Recovery and Recovery Capital: Aligning Measurement with Theory and Practice

H. Harrington Cleveland, Timothy R. Brick, Kyler S. Knapp, and Julie M. Croff

Great efforts have been made to understand *who* is in successful recovery from substance use disorders (SUD) – that is, to understand the characteristics of individuals who are successful in recovery. Recovery is an ongoing and dynamic process; it is possible to be successful, relapse, and then again be successful. A focus on recovery as an ongoing process suggests that understanding *when* recovery is successful for each individual and *how* processes that sustain recovery may change over time may be more important than understanding *who* is successful in a moment. In this chapter, we argue that successful recovery is a dynamic process comprised of more components than abstinence. We propose that researchers interested in addiction recovery should adopt measurement, modeling, and intervention paradigms that match the multicomponent environmental and within-person nature of recovery. Specifically, researchers should adopt measurement that captures the dynamics of change within the process of recovery for different individuals across many timescales and contexts; that utilizes the concept of *recovery capital*, the set of resources that support recovery; and that models the ongoing transactions between recovery status and recovery capital. In Sect. 1, we set out the importance of recovery and examine recent definitions of the term. In Sect. 2, we define recovery capital and discuss current strategies and future directions for understanding it and its interactions with the process of recovery. Section 3 examines current approaches to measuring recovery and contrasts this with the definitions of recovery reviewed in Sect. 1. Section 4 describes measurement approaches for modeling recovery capital that

H. H. Cleveland (✉) · T. R. Brick · K. S. Knapp
Department of Human Development and Family Studies, The Pennsylvania State University, University Park, PA, USA
e-mail: hhc10@psu.edu

J. M. Croff
National Center for Wellness and Recovery, Oklahoma State University Center for Health Sciences, Tulsa, OK, USA

J. M. Croff, J. Beaman (eds.), *Family Resilience and Recovery from Opioids and Other Addictions*, Emerging Issues in Family and Individual Resilience,
https://doi.org/10.1007/978-3-030-56958-7_6

contribute to the maintenance of recovery well-being. To make our argument more concrete, Sect. 5 describes recovery support programs that are tailored for different populations and different contexts, setting out how the dynamics of recovery and recovery capital might be assessed within these programs.

1 Recovery: What Is It?

"Recovery" is a nontechnical term used in both nonprofessional and professional SUD settings to describe a state of health and functioning that follows the cessation of addictive substance use, typically involving abstinence from use (White 1998). Over the last two decades, recognition of the importance of recovery has led several academic, professional, and government organizations to develop formal definitions for recovery. Several of these definitions are provided in Table 6.1. At the core of most of these definitions is the idea that although abstinence from the addictive substance may be required, recovery also requires addressing underlying causes of SUD and improving individual well-being beyond nonuse or remission. Similarly, the ongoing nature of recovery is evident in definitions describing recovery as a "state…of health" (ASAM 2005) and a "lifestyle" (Betty Ford Institute Consensus Panel 2007; see Table 6.1, which provides the same definitions presented in Kelly

Table 6.1 Prominent addiction recovery definitions

Source	Year	Definition
American Society of Addiction Medicine (ASAM)	2005	A patient is in a "state of recovery" when he or she has reached a state of physical and psychological health such that his/her abstinence from dependency-producing drugs is complete and comfortable
Betty Ford Institute Consensus Panel	2006	A voluntarily maintained lifestyle characterized by sobriety, personal health, and citizenship
Center for Substance Abuse Treatment	2005	Recovery from alcohol and drug problems is a process of change through which an individual achieves abstinence and improved health, wellness, and quality of life
SAMHSA	2011	Recovery from mental disorders and substance use disorders is a process of change through which individuals improve their health and wellness, live a self-directed life, and strive to reach their full potential
Scottish Government	2008	A process through which an individual is enabled to move on from their problem drug use, towards a drug-free life as an active and contributing member of society
UK Drug Policy Commission	2008	The process of recovery from problematic substance use is characterized by voluntarily sustained control over substance use which maximizes health and well-being and participation in the rights, roles, and responsibilities of society

and Hoeppner 2015) and the dynamic nature repeatedly reasserted by descriptions of recovery as a "process" or a "process of change" (e.g., CSAT 2005; SAMHSA 2011). Although abstinence or sobriety is a feature of most definitions, so too are physical and psychological health, wellness, quality of life, and societal engagement. The overall sense is that recovery must be understood as a transformational dynamic process that unfolds over time and encompasses development and maintenance of a broad set of behavioral, cognitive, social, and physical characteristics. Consistent with this broader conceptualization, Kaskutas et al. (2014) note that the Big Book of AA describes a program of recovery and that abstinence requires developing a "new way of living." Given these definitions, we will argue later in this chapter that measurement of recovery should not only go beyond monitoring nonuse to capture other factors related to health and well-being but that it should be undertaken in a way that sheds light on the dynamic processes that underlie and constitute recovery as it is lived.

Conceptually, Kelly and Hoeppner (2015) raise several questions that serve as an excellent guide to highlight the ambiguities present in the definitions presented in Table 6.1. First, *is recovery a single common process?* If so, recovery across individuals would essentially be the same. If not, individuals with qualitatively different versions of recovery could still be equally engaged in the process of recovery. Second, *what place does personal health and wellness have in recovery*? Definitions put forth by CSAT (2005) and SAMHSA (2011; see Table 6.1) both describe recovery as a process of change for which the outcome is individuals improving their health and achieving improved health. In contrast, other definitions situate well-being as part of recovery, rather than an outcome. For example, the Betty Ford Institute's (2007) definition lists personal health as a characteristic of recovery. Similarly, ASAM states that a "state of recovery" is a "state of physical and psychological health." These definitions' different orientations toward well-being create uncertainty regarding whether improved well-being is an outcome or end goal of recovery or a component part intrinsic to the larger process of recovery.

Third, *what is the role of civic engagement or engagement with others generally*? Definitions from the Betty Ford Institute (2007) and both the Scottish government and the UK Drug Policy Commission (2008) include civic engagement, participating in or contributing to society as part of recovery, but these are not included in the other definitions. Although there may be good reasons to believe that isolation may threaten many individuals' recoveries, existing definitions do not completely align regarding whether a recovery built on solitude is possible.

Taken together, these definitions exhibit ambiguity concerning the homogeneity vs. heterogeneity of the recovery process across individuals, contexts, and time. Moreover, there are also ambiguities around how to consider those aspects of recovery that go beyond nonuse and are more focused on thriving and striving to improve one's condition, as well as the relationships between individuals, their recovery, and the broader society.

2 Recovery Capital

The construct of "recovery capital" provides a framework for examining resources that support the process of recovery. This concept is relatively new – at least formally – in the field of recovery research (Granfield and Cloud 1999, 2004). On the most basic level, recovery capital includes all resources someone has access to and the capacity of the individual to use these resources to support their recovery: including social, physical, human, and cultural capital. Similar to recovery itself, recovery capital is also complex and dynamic.

In defining recovery capital, Granfield and Cloud (1999, 2004) distinguish between social and physical capital. Social capital is the sum of resources that people have as a result of their relationships and includes both support from and obligations to groups to which they belong. Physical capital includes tangible assets such as property and money that may increase recovery options, such as being able to pay for better treatment options (e.g., medication-assisted treatments for opioid and alcohol use disorders) and opportunities to access posttreatment settings (e.g., supportive recovery housing). Physical capital and social capital can mutually influence each other. For example, an individual might use physical resources (e.g., money) to move away from networks of users and seek out opportunities to add recovering friends to their social networks. Alternatively, an individual might rely on a network of friends to help make ends meet financially. Despite this mutual influence, the two are still conceptually independent. Being financially able to move to a new town may create opportunities to add recovering or supportive friends to one's social network, but it does not directly create or maintain those relationships.

Human capital includes education, skills, positive health, aspirations, hopes, "grit," and other personal resources that enable individuals to prosper. Education is a particularly important aspect of human capital that supports recovery, because education increases the potential for productive and professional engagement. Similarly, interpersonal skills can have clear impact on someone's ability to build and maintain relationships that may provide additional support.

Cultural capital includes the values, beliefs, and attitudes that link individuals to prosocial norms and identities and aid in reconceptualizing oneself – both within the recovery community and within general society. This reconceptualization is closely tied to the psychological construct of mattering, an important aspect of self-concept, which defines how human beings have a need to be significant to others, attend to others, and to serve as a resource to others (Elliott et al. 2004). Indeed, this concept interacts with the process and definitions of recovery presented above. Negative self-concept is a defining characteristic of substance use disorder (Dumont & Vamos 1975), and reconceptualization is a critically important hallmark of transition to recovery dependent on cultural capital and interaction with others.

The analogy of *capital* is an important one. Physical capital (e.g., net worth) can take many forms: a person might have money in the form of cash or as in investment; these can be applied in different ways. Cash has a tremendous influence on a person's ability to purchase goods or to deal with a sudden debt. By contrast, investments might not be immediately useful to purchase goods, but can provide benefits over the longer term. In the same way, recovery capital may take on very different forms, each of which may be more or less suited to a given person, context, and time, and each of which may provide benefits that only become evident at different points in time. This variability makes the consistent measurement of recovery capital and modeling its effects on recovery more difficult than might be immediately obvious.

2.1 Relationship Between Recovery and Recovery Capital

The relationship between recovery and recovery capital is characterized by a reciprocal process. On one hand, such relationships can lead to beneficial trajectories with increased capital sparking improved recovery, which allows the individual to accumulate more capital. On the other hand, an individual who faces repeated recovery challenges may quickly burn through recovery capital (e.g., by overburdening social supporters), each time leading to fewer resources available for the next challenge. During active addiction, the reciprocal process between an individual's own state of wellbeing, or lack thereof, and their increasingly damaged social relationships may contribute to what has been referred to as "rock bottom." Variance in individual capital is present from before the onset of substance use disorder through the recovery process, resulting in differential success in the process of recovery. The following examples set out different ways in which recovery capital may support or undercut recovery.

Some individuals with substance use addictions have substantial finances, insurance policies, opportunities for higher quality and longer treatment and post-treatment care, and the ability to move away from their old set of using peers to form new peer groups of nonusers and individuals in recovery. By contrast, others do not have the same resources for treatment and may be tied via financial concerns to a single job and location and may therefore find it difficult to avoid social groups with substance-using peers, and potential cascades of triggers to use, negative affect, and cravings. Not all differences in recovery capital are external to the individual or even stable over time. For example, individuals who are committed to their recoveries may be more likely to attend support group meetings and develop supportive social networks. These investments can create more resources for individuals to draw upon over time as they do the daily work of maintaining well-being and/or dealing with acute threats to their recoveries. Conversely, an individual who does not invest in their recovery will likely have less recovery capital to draw upon when needed.

The observation that recovery and recovery capital are integrated and interactive is not unique to this chapter. For example, the central idea of Kelly and Hoeppner's (2015) proposed biaxial formulation of recovery is that as remission becomes more stable and longer-term, there are (generally) improvements to recovery capital. Similarly, the more recovery capital is accrued, in the form of intrapersonal capabilities and interpersonal support, the more likely remission will continue. Accordingly, growth along these axes (i.e., remission and recovery capital) is linked in a reciprocal fashion. Kelly and Hoeppner (2015) propose that the link between them is mediated by ability to cope with stressors and triggers. Consistent with our view, Kelly and Hoeppner emphasize that recovery is dynamic and involves changing relationships between stressors and individual capacities. The centrality of the transactions among people's characteristics, triggers, and resources to our understanding of recovery capital underscores the need for methods that capture these within-person processes.

3 Measurement Approaches for Studying Recovery

If recovery is multifaceted and dynamic, it follows that measurement strategies should be implemented that are designed to capture dynamic and multifaceted processes. Kaskutas et al. (2014) empirically assessed several recovery domains, focusing on both discovering the most common specific elements of recovery and identifying differences among the unique pathways taken by individuals. Their study utilized 47 items drawn from the World Health Organization (WHO) scales and recruited participants from diverse recovery settings. Results revealed four defined domains of recovery: abstinence in recovery (i.e., no use/misuse of drugs), essentials of recovery (i.e., responding to mistakes and negative feelings), enriched recovery (i.e., contributing to family/society), and spirituality of recovery (i.e., being grateful). These four domains cover similar ground as those proposed by SAMHSA in 2011, which include purpose (similar to spirituality), community (similar to enriched recovery), and health (related to both abstinence and negative feelings), and therefore provide data-driven support for SAMHSA's domains. However, the Kaskutas et al. (2014) study also revealed that some of these unique elements, such as essentials of recovery, were especially important to some subgroups of people in recovery. They also found differences in engagement in these distinct strategies between individuals, varying by characteristics such as experience in treatment and time in recovery. Their findings suggest that these four primary domains may vary in importance across individuals, contexts, and time in recovery.

Differences in factor scores across contextual and individual variables highlight the need for measurement that can assess differences both between individuals and contexts and across time within a single individual. Each of the four factors identified by Kaskutas et al. (2014) may not only differ across people (e.g., some individuals are better able to deal with mistakes and negative feelings than others), but they may also vary within people by context (e.g., individuals being better able to deal with mistakes and negative feelings within some spaces or social groups than in others), and time (e.g., individuals being better able to deal with mistakes and negative feelings on same days than on others).

Behavioral response to protect and build recovery will vary by timescale. The relevant timescale for linkages between intrapersonal states, such as craving or negative mood, and behavioral reactions, and subsequent outcomes, might be hours or minutes. Behaviors might result in release of endorphins and improved sleep, therein reinforcing a positive behavior cascade which started from a negative emotion. By contrast, civic engagement requires repeated behavioral engagements to lead to positive results. The result of civic engagement may be less helpful in addressing short-term negative affect, but may strengthen a person's recovery identity and reduce risk of relapse in the coming months and years. The experiences of dealing with negative emotion, and subsequent engagement in positive behaviors, may, over time, reduce the strength of substance craving, as new behavioral patterns take hold. During this transition, engagement in long-term outcomes, like civic engagement, may increase in importance for sustained recovery. The recovery process requires engagement across domains, which yield benefits at different timescales. Therefore, it is necessary for measurement approaches to capture engagement across domains at different times as well.

4 Measurement Approaches for Studying Recovery Capital and Its Relationship to Recovery

Although studies assessing broadly defined views of recovery itself are sparse, the measurement of recovery capital has received greater attention, with a focus on understanding its different domains. A recent systematic review of the literature by Hennessy (2017) found 35 unique studies examining recovery capital, with sample sizes ranging from 4 to 703 participants. Findings from this review indicated that recovery capital has been studied in a range of diverse populations, yet conceptualization of the key domains and quantitative measurement have been inconsistent. For example, the first attempt to measure recovery capital (Sterling et al. 2008) focused on personal and social capital with a heavy emphasis on spirituality, but did not demonstrate ability to predict recovery success across participants. Another instrument, the Recovery Capital Questionnaire (RCQ; Burns and Marks 2013), assesses four domains: social, physical, human, and community capital. Both of these tools showed measurement validity but have not been utilized in applied contexts.

The Assessment of Recovery Capital (ARC; Groshkova et al. 2013) and other measures subsequently developed from it changed this trend, being used in applied studies of recovery focused on targets besides scale development. The ARC assesses a variety of domains, including substance use and sobriety, psychological and physical health, community involvement, social support, and more. However, rather than providing evidence of multiple domains, principal components analysis suggested that a single-component structure provided the best fit to the data. Vilsaint et al. (2017) drew from the 50-item pool of the ARC to test a reduced version of the ARC assessing a single unified dimension: the Brief Assessment of Recovery Capital (BARC-10). Results revealed that this new measure demonstrated internal consistency, concurrent and predictive validity, and measurement invariance across location and gender, suggesting that it is a strong measure to distinguish differences in recovery capital at a between-persons level.

The REC-CAP was designed as a broader tool that incorporates the ARC as one of its component parts, alongside other measures assessing recovery goals, engagement, and motivation, to create a more holistic assessment of recovery capital (Best et al. 2016). The instrument is primarily intended to identify strengths and barriers to recovery by capturing individuals' amounts of personal, social, and community recovery capital. Unlike other measures such as the ARC, which are largely used for research purposes, the REC-CAP is designed for use in various recovery settings for monitoring of progress by both the participant and professional or nonprofessional staff and can inform recovery planning over time (Best et al. 2016, 2017).

Each of these measures (with the possible exception of the REC-CAP) is validated using data collected at a between-persons level. That is, they assess each person at a single point in time and cannot distinguish differences between people from differences in, for example, stage of recovery. As a result, these measures are likely to focus on those aspects that differentiate people from each other – called *interindividual variability* in the literature. Future directions should include measurement of changes in capital within individuals to assess whether capital can increase, decrease, or change form over time throughout an individual's recovery journey, and the study of interindividual variability misses those changes. This second set of variability is termed *intraindividual variability* (Nesselroade & Ram 2004). Measures that focus on interindividual differences will often miss crucial factors that matter within a given person's development (Molenaar 2004). Therefore, efforts are needed to develop, test, and utilize measures that assess recovery capital longitudinally in ecologically valid ways (e.g., measuring it in context as it is unfolding rather than only in the lab or at one sitting using retrospective recall).

Modern technological tools have begun to provide a means of assessing this type of intraindividual change. New approaches to measurement, referred to collectively as "slice of life methods" (Smyth et al. 2017), focus on collecting intensive longitudinal data about a single individual across time while they live their everyday lives. Two common approaches are the *daily diary* method and *ecological momentary assessment.* Daily diary methods ask participants to provide a single report each day describing their experiences throughout the day (Bolger et al. 2003). These once-a-day reports require a relatively small burden on the part of the participant but provide a clear view of the within-person changes and patterns that occur on a day-to-day level.

Within-day processes may still, however, be important to recovery and recovery capital. For example, negative social interactions at midday may have a detrimental impact on later day mood and craving (see Cleveland and Harris 2010). Conversely, positive support from a friend in recovery, an engagement in social recovery capital, may increase the salience of an individual's own recovery commitment for that day and reduce the impact of a negative social experience on end of day mood or craving. *Ecological momentary assessment* approaches use technological tools (frequently smartphones, in modern studies) to request feedback from participants several times a day (Stone and Shiffman 1994). These studies permit researchers to examine differences in recovery, as well as recovery capital within and between days. Applying mixed-effects and multilevel models (Pritikin et al. 2017; Oravecz and Brick 2019) to these types of data allows researchers to identify the phenomena that matter at different times and contexts for a single individual, as well as those that differentiate individuals from one another. In the case of the former, for example, an individual might be strongly affected by negative social experiences when he/she has low positive mood, but not when that individual is experiencing high amounts of positive mood. EMA approaches also allow researchers to investigate between-person differences in such within-person processes. For example, some people may be highly reactive to negative social experiences, leading to strong impacts on mood and craving from only a single interaction, while another might show much less reactivity. Even more interesting, this reactivity may also change within-person across time, with different patterns of change for each individual. These patterns may be driven by the process of recovery itself or may be in response to outside factors, such as social interactions, current location or environment, and the accessibility of support services.

5 Where Recovery Happens: Recovery Support Services

Most conventional research on recovery has begun by searching for metrics indicating the success of SUD treatment in a context like a residential rehabilitation facility, or rather, following release from such treatment. Yet, the adoption of recovery as an ongoing process has driven two paradigmatic shifts: first, the move from a focus on symptoms/pathology to a wellness framework, and second, the move from a perspective that recovery is the aftermath of treatment to a perspective that recovery is an ongoing process that requires chronic/continuing care (White 2006; Laudet 2011). These paradigm shifts also suggest a movement from measurement of recovery in terms of fixed treatment outcomes (such as relapse within the first 90 days of completing treatment) to measurement of metrics indicative of positive growth and continued maintenance. This shift in conceptualizing the measurement of recovery is not only due to the multifaceted and individualized nature of recovery but also reflects the reality that many who are engaged in recovery do so without treatment (Sobell et al. 2000). Thus, someone being actively involved in recovery does not assume they have graduated from treatment. Indeed, a nationally representative study by Kelly and colleagues found that only 28% of people who report being in recovery went to any form of formal treatment (Kelly et al. 2017). Even within the 28% whose path to recovery involves formal treatment, only half did so via residential treatment, which is undoubtedly the most commonly studied setting. More commonly, recovery is found via involvement in mutual help support groups or the growing number of recovery centers and sober living environments, many of which have only been available in the last 15–20 years (Kelly et al. 2017).

Accordingly, research efforts must explore contexts beyond formal treatment settings. In order to generate lasting effects, it is critical to understand the recovery support programs that provide the support necessary for short-term recovery maintenance and the opportunities to develop other aspects of recovery capital necessary for building long-term recovery. This point is well made by Kelly et al. (2017), who point out that in contrast to the great volume of treatment center work, there is relatively little work on recovery support services, such as collegiate recovery communities (see Cleveland et al. 2010) and recovery housing (see Polcin and Borkman 2008; Jason and Ferrari 2010).

Below we first distinguish between professional and peer-delivered recovery support services and then review two different types of programs that support recovery in different settings: Collegiate Recovery Communities and Recovery Housing. Broader reviews of such programs exist in other places (see Laudet and Humphreys 2013). Our purpose here is twofold: (1) set out different types of programs and contexts in a fashion that illustrates the differences in recovery capital provided by these programs targeting different populations and different contexts and (2) discuss how research and evaluation of these different program settings can be tailored to capture the dynamic transactions between individuals and the aspects of recovery capital that are offered by and can be cultivated within these programs.

5.1 Distinguishing Between Professional and Peer-Delivered Recovery Support Services

Recovery support programs typically help individuals address a hierarchy of needs that could adversely affect recovery. These needs are greatest in the beginning of the recovery process and addressing them creates the scaffolding on which recovery capital is built. The hierarchy of needs addressed are most notably in the domains of employment, education, social relationships, and housing (Laudet and Humphreys 2013). Recovery support services can be provided by either professionals or peers. Professional recovery support services frequently consist of recovery management checkups (RMC) that monitor clients' status, address relapse risks, and link clients to services during gaps in employment. Staff often use motivational interviewing techniques to help clients recognize relapse risks and further their engagement activities. These services both link individuals to recovery capital and help them develop the tools to access recovery capital resources.

Peer-delivered recovery support services are defined as the process of giving and receiving nonprofessional, nonclinical assistance to achieve long-term recovery (Bassuk et al. 2016). This support is provided by peers with experiential knowledge who are in recovery themselves and serve as both models and advisors for others in recovery (Borkman 1999). These individuals can be either paid or volunteer, and their qualifications for providing support vary across settings. Some have required durations of drug/alcohol abstinence to qualify for peer recovery coach credentials. For example, Tennessee's Certified Recovery Specialist requires individuals be in recovery and take 40 h of dedicated training; Pennsylvania requires 75 h of training. The services that are provided are delivered in various forms (e.g., one-on-one services, group settings) and in different contexts, such as recovery community centers, faith-based institutions, jails and prisons, social service centers, and addiction treatment agencies. This support will include helping the individual set recovery goals and develop and maintain a recovery plan. The supporting peer can connect the individual with recovery resources in the community and serve as an advocate for the individual in these settings. In other words, peers are simultaneously recovery capital themselves and guides for individuals regarding how to identify and cultivate recovery capital.

Research protocols within these settings should be tailored to address the specific recovery capital needs of the recovering population being studied and the specific sources of recovery support that are provided by the program setting, whether formal or informal. Specifically, the frequency of different recovery-supportive (as well as recovery-challenging) events should be considered. For example, an individual may have daily Twelve-Step meetings, weekly scheduled meetings with a recovery specialist, and numerous – but unscheduled and irregularly spaced – interactions with a sponsor. In professional-led settings, such as MAT outpatient settings with counseling, protocols could assess the craving experiences of the patients as well as the situations that are linked to higher or lower levels of craving. Accordingly, measurement paradigms should ensure that recovery metrics are assessed frequently enough to capture their variability across time and to understand the events that are supportive and detrimental to recovery.

5.1.1 Collegiate Recovery Communities

Some recovery support programs are highly tailored to specific populations and settings. A prime example is Collegiate Recovery Communities (CRC). These programs directly support the recovery needs of populations engaged in higher education. Education can directly contribute to recovery capital by increasing opportunities for employment and meaningful engagement in society, both of which can help promote recovery. CRCs also address the recovery needs of their participants in a developmentally targeted fashion. One of the difficulties younger (i.e., teen and young adult) individuals in recovery face is the lack of fit between the conventional mutual help group context and their own experiences (see Russell, Cleveland, and Wiebe 2010). CRCs are tailored to the developmental challenges being negotiated by these young individuals generally, and the specific challenges they encounter as they try to maintain recovery in their educational settings.

Like most recovery support, CRCs are generally informed by Twelve-Step tenets. Their general goal is to provide supportive communities that deliver developmentally appropriate support for their members. CRCs conventionally provide a drop-in center, where members can spend time between classes. The communities are supported by program staff, who provide relapse prevention and life skills workshops as well as work with members of the community to organize sober recreational activities and service opportunities (Harris, Baker, and Cleveland 2010; Laudet and Humphreys 2013).

CRCs differ substantially in terms of size (from only a few to over 100 members) and in the characteristics of their members, such as demographics, time in recovery, and drug of choice. They also differ in the scale of the role of program staff. In all cases the staff provides support for the community, although program staff play a more direct supervisory and even therapeutic role in some cases. The degree to which communities differ in direct vs. indirect role of staff also manifests in whether and how they provide and regulate recovery housing. Some programs provide on-campus housing including on-site clinical professionals. Others provide recovery housing on campus, but do not provide professional staff to supervise residents. These housing contexts may have a senior member of the community act as lead resident. Still others do not provide housing at all but work to match members of the community together as housemates in private rentals. Still other programs provide no assistance with housing. Full descriptions of CRCs are available in Laudet et al. (2015) and Cleveland et al. (2007). Program variability in size, average length of recovery, and level of support needs to be considered when attempting to understand how recovery develops and is maintained within these settings.

5.1.2 Recovery Housing

Recovery residences are residential self-help communal living facilities that contribute to continued abstinence by providing a network of others who share abstinence goals and creating conditions to gain employment skills (Gómez et al. 2014). These residences also encourage social support, civic engagement, and physical health and well-being. These residences are open to a wider range of individuals than those served by CRCs, whose reach is limited to individuals who are able to pursue higher education and have the financial ability to do so. Recovery residences recruit from either community treatment or criminal justice agencies and require abstinence, mutual aid, meeting attendance, getting and keeping employment, and contributing to the common upkeep and well-being of the residence (Cano et al. 2017). These residences provide both housing and stability for individuals embarking on the recovery process outside of traditional treatment centers. One of the critical aspects of these programs is that they provide conditions for individuals to gain useful employment skills (Gómez et al. 2014). Better employment helps support recovery in several ways, including helping residents redevelop purpose and identity as well as connecting them to the world beyond themselves and their immediate focus on recovery itself (see Burrow and Hill 2011). Accordingly, employment can provide "bridging social capital," a resource that is critical for avoiding social isolation and supporting long-term recovery. For more information on recovery houses – as well as Oxford houses, which are self-governing recovery homes – and their impact on recovery, see Cano et al. (2017), Polcin et al. (2010), Jason et al. (2006), and Olson et al. (2009).

5.1.3 Measurement in CRCs and Recovery Housing

Research conducted within CRCs should assess both daily interactions within drop-in centers as well as the (presumably less frequent) contact with staff. Assessments should also aim to capture social interactions among members of the community outside of the center and across the day. The nesting of these groups within the broader university community means that non-SUD comparison groups can be assembled that share a common set of contexts. Program events, such as recovery workshops and alternative sober social events, could provide excellent "natural experiments" by assessing differences between participants and nonparticipants over the time period following the event, as well as examining the impact of attending these events on the well-being of participants immediately following engaging in these events. Future research should consider both the impact of program and social experiences on individuals' well-being and the influence of individuals' mood on their frequency of engagement with formal program events and interactions with community members.

Studies focused on recovery houses may have unique opportunities to study the influences of social forces and individual identity on (and of) recovery. The focus of these residences on identity, employment, and social support provide an excellent means to examine the way that overlapping spheres of social influence (e.g., within the recovery house, at work, and in the greater community) may interact with each individuals' recovery identity over time. Studies of these communities are also well-suited to examine questions of community involvement and civic engagement.

6 Implications

6.1 Implications for Understanding Family Resilience

As has been described in detail in other chapters in this book, the recovery process has implications beyond the individuals in recovery (Bradshaw et al. 2020; Hays-Grudo et al. 2020; Ciciolla et al. 2020). Measurement of the recovery process, and the context that supports that process, requires inclusion of social systems. Among individuals with high recovery capital at the start of the process, these social systems may include immediate family. Immediate family systems may be conceptualized as parents, spouses/partners, or children of individuals with substance use disorders. Just as likely for individuals who experienced childhood trauma (Hays-Grudo et al. 2020), family systems may be trusted and loved aunts, uncles, or other individuals who are part of a made-family. Regardless of relationship, the substance use disorder affects and destabilizes the whole family unit. The resilience of the family unit aligns with the recovery capital of the individual and includes social, physical, human, and cultural capital.

For researchers interested in understanding family and individual resilience in the context of recovery, there are many methodological issues to consider. Interpersonal assessments within family systems may improve understanding of context, time, and individual characteristics on recovery and recovery capital. However, these intensive measurements may be burdensome to participants and their families – stopping one's day four to six times to answer surveys is simply a lot of effort. It is important for researchers interested in this approach, therefore, to carefully select the questions that need to be asked and to take care to balance the scientific gain of each question or survey against the burden for participants (Brick et al. 2020). Particularly within the context of measuring multiple family members, it is important to minimize the conflict such measurement can cause within the family system. Within the context of treatment for substance use disorder, our research group has implemented a 12-day assessment protocol with four assessments per day at early morning, late morning, early afternoon, and evening by carefully scheduling data collection times to avoid treatment activities, keeping surveys short, and providing flexible response windows.

A second concern of particular importance in recovery settings is the requirement for privacy. The intensive data that can be collected with smartphones (e.g., GPS, heart rate, self-report, social context, etc.) adds a significant risk to participants if data are publicly disclosed. Especially in recovery settings where some patients may have social and family networks that are unaware of their prior use, special care must be taken to ensure that privacy is maintained. While work is ongoing to create privacy-preserving methods of data collection and analysis (see, e.g., Boker et al. 2015; Snoke et al. 2018), current best practices involve ensuring proper data security, limiting data collection to only what is needed, avoiding personally identifying data collection whenever possible, and removing any remaining identifiers at the first opportunity.

Several other tools exist to assist researchers. *Burst designs*, which use short, intensive bursts of measurement interspersed with times of less intense measurement, can capture moment-to-moment variability within a person and the way it changes across time during recovery without overburdening the participant with long bursts of intensive measurement (see, e.g., Ram and Diehl 2015). For example, a study could follow individuals from when they begin recovery until a year later, but reduce burden by using four 21-day bursts of data collection at months 1, 4, 8, and 12 to capture both within-person dynamics of recovery (assessed with the intensive bursts) and how these dynamics shift across the year (by comparing patterns across the bursts). Finally, passive measurement tools, such as wearable heart rate wristbands, can be used to identify moments of risk (Osotsi et al. 2020), stress (Hovsepian et al. 2015), and craving (Chatterjee et al. 2016). Perhaps more importantly, these tools can be used to deliver targeted assessment to capture both the participant's perspective and the more objective measures of stress and craving (Bertz et al. 2018; Brick et al. 2020).

6.2 *Promising Applications*

Best et al.'s (2016) qualitative evidence suggests that opportunities to build bridging social capital vis-à-vis links to the local community beyond those in recovery is an important aspect of recovery programs. A new and compelling program for recovery support has been introduced in Blackpool, England. The Jobs, Friends, and Housing program is a social enterprise supported by the local law enforcement in Lancashire, UK. In addition to providing access to recovery activities in the evenings and on weekends, the program provides training and employment in the construction industry for people in recovery. The recovering individuals who are part of the program work to build or renovate houses and either sell them for profit to be reinvested in the Jobs, Friends, and Houses enterprise or rent them out as recovery housing for others in recovery. Building recovery housing links members' labor to "giving back" to the community and helps them develop social capital and extend their lives beyond the world of recovery.

The methodological challenges and opportunities presented by evaluating professionally staffed recovery houses, Oxford Houses, and programs similar to Jobs, Friends, and Housing are intriguing. These programs are designed to facilitate a deep transition in individuals' lives. They are designed to do so via providing important components of recovery capital for individuals to access, benefit from, and further develop. Thus, evaluations of these programs that are primarily focused on how many of their individual program attendees or community members are abstinent after finite periods of time, such as 30 days, 6 months, or a year, are missing an opportunity to consider the dynamic social transactions through which recovery and recovery capital are built. Rather, it is critical to understand the degree and quality of their social interactions, with whom these interactions take place, where they take place, and the value or lack thereof that individuals gain from these interactions. The data collections and analyses need to align timescales with the dynamic nature of social transactions and their impact on individuals' well-being. For example, do the recovery seminars/workshops provided by collegiate recovery programs or recovery houses have short-term impacts on the daily well-being or recovery identity of community members? Do program experiences contribute to changes in the characteristics of social networks (e.g., the number of abstinent individuals within a social network) or – perhaps more importantly – the strategic and timely use of members' recovery support social networks? Just as technology can be used to assess the dynamic nature of recovery itself and recovery capital, it can also be deployed to assess how and when program components affect these processes.

7 Conclusion and Future Directions

Recovery is a continual process that requires ongoing change in a person's social, cognitive, and behavioral patterns to thrive during sustained abstinence from substance use and requires a tremendous amount of recovery capital. Treatment can begin the process of abstinence and provide some small amount of recovery capital, but falls far short of the capacities needed for sustained recovery success. This mismatch between what recovery needs and what treatment alone provides is consistent with the high percentage of posttreatment relapse as well as the high proportion of individuals who find recovery without treatment. This observation does not suggest that treatment providers have nothing to offer. In contrast, treatment providers are often the best positioned to guide individuals to the recovery support they need (Best and Laudet 2010). Nonetheless, it is clear that treatment alone is not sufficient, and research priorities that disproportionately focus on treatment are misguided. What we propose is a research agenda that focuses on a multifaceted view of recovery and meaningfully considers that recovery is a within-person process that varies across time, individual, and context. To match this complexity, methods and analyses will have to capture and consider within- and between-person variability in these aspects. Further, more work is needed to study recovery and its reciprocal relationship with recovery capital in the contexts in which recovery occurs and across the various timescales on which recovery is built and maintained. These studies will have to capture not only the multifaceted nature of recovery and the complexity of within-person processes and how they shift across time, but also the meaningful heterogeneity in which recovery capital is accumulated and spent across different contexts (Breakout Box 6.1).

Breakout Box 6.1. Focus on Experience

I'll never forget the day that my brother told me about his drug addiction. He was 16. I came home one day from school and he was waiting for me in the family room. He had tears streaming down his face as he told me that he needed my help. He'd been using crack and he didn't want to tell my parents. He cried and slapped his head saying that he just wanted to kill himself. Once my mother found out, she made arrangements for him to leave the state to live with a relative to get away from the drugs. He left and things only got worse. He began using opioids and eventually was arrested for a DUI. After he served his time, he moved back home. Things were good for a few months. We were very hopeful. We thought that things had gotten bad enough for him that he would never go back to it. But then his behavior changed. He didn't want to be around. He found excuses to leave family parties early. He started stealing from my parents and had brought drug dealers to their home. I feel that we were slow to catch on. I don't know why we didn't approach him earlier. I think we all wanted to believe that he had changed and that he was finally going to be safe and happy, but things couldn't have been worse. He went to jail again, this time for 60 days. It was a relief. At least we knew he was safe, that he wasn't somewhere overdosing. Part of his probation terms included completing an outpatient drug program. He has but I still expect him to end up in jail again or overdosing. When my mother calls, I often worry it's to tell me he is dead. But there are times when I really feel hope for him. He is more open about his addiction than he has been. I can see a change in his desire to change. Even when he messes up, I think he tries to get back on track quicker.

– Elizabeth – sister of a recovering opioid addict

Glossary of Terms

Daily diary participants provide a single report each day describing their experiences throughout the day to track day-to-day level changes or patterns (Bolger et al. 2003)

Ecological momentary assessment approaches that use technological tools (frequently smartphones, in modern studies) to request feedback from participants several times a day with the goal of collecting information about experiences in the context in which they occur close in time to the experiences

Intraindividual change change within an individual

Recovery nontechnical term used in both nonprofessional and professional SUD settings to describe a state of health and functioning that follows the cessation of addictive substance use, typically involving abstinence from use (White 1998); a dynamic process

Recovery capital includes all resources someone has access to and the capacity of the individual to use these resources to support their recovery including social, physical, human, and cultural capital

Recovery support services services that support recovery, provided by either professionals or peers

References

American Society of Addiction Medicine. (2005). Public policy statement on the state of recovery, Chevy Chase.

Bassuk, E. L., Hanson, J., Greene, R. N., Richard, M., & Laudet, A. (2016). Peer-delivered recovery support services for addictions in the United States: A systematic review. *Journal of Substance Abuse Treatment, 63*, 1–9. https://doi.org/10.1016/j.jsat.2016.01.003.

Bertz, J. W., Epstein, D. H., & Preston, K. L. (2018). Combining ecological momentary assessment with objective, ambulatory measures of behavior and physiology in substance-use research. *Addictive Behaviors, 83*, 5–17. https://doi.org/10.1016/j.addbeh.2017.11.027.

Best, D., & Laudet, A. B. (2010). *The potential of recovery capital*. RSA Projects. Retrieved from www.ukdpc.org.uk/

Best, D., Beswick, T., Hodgkins, S., & Idle, M. (2016). Recovery, ambitions, and aspirations: An exploratory project to build a recovery community by generating a skilled recovery workforce. *Alcoholism Treatment Quarterly, 34*(1), 3–14. https://doi.org/10.1080/07347324.2016.1113105.

Best, D., Irving, J., Collinson, B., Andersson, C., & Edwards, M. (2017). Recovery networks and community connections: Identifying connection needs and community linkage opportunities in early recovery populations. https://doi.org/10.1080/07347324.2016.1256718.

Boker, S. M., Brick, T. R., von Oertzen, T., Estabrook, R., Pritikin, J. N., Hunter, M. D., Maes, H. H., & Neale, M. C. (2015). Maintained individual data distributed likelihood estimation (MIDDLE). *Multivariate Behavioral Research, 50*(6), 706–720. https://doi.org/10.1080/00273171.2015.1094387.

Bolger, N., Davis, A., & Rafaeli, E. (2003). Diary methods: Capturing life as it is lived. *Annual Review of Psychology, 54*(1), 579–616. https://doi.org/10.1146/annurev.psych.54.101601.145030.

Bradshaw, S., Shumway, S., & Kimball, T. (2020). Associations between SUD in the family, PFC functioning, and codependency: Importance of family member recovery. In J. Croff &

J. Beaman (Eds.), *Family resilience and recovery: Opioids and other addictions*. Springer. Manuscript submitted for publication.

Brick, T. R., Mundie, J., Weaver, J., Fraleigh, R., & Oravecz, Z. (2020). Wear-IT: Low-burden Mobile monitoring and intervention through real-time analysis. *Journal of Medical Internet Research (JMIR): Formative Research*. https://doi.org/10.2196/16072.

Borkman, T. (1999). *Understanding self-help/mutual aid: Experiential learning in the commons*. New Brunswick, NJ: Rutgers University Press.

Burrow, A. L., & Hill, P. L. (2011). Purpose as a form of identity capital for positive youth adjustment. *Developmental Psychology, 47*(4), 1196–1206. https://doi.org/10.1037/a0023818.

Burns, J., & Marks, D. (2013). Can recovery capital predict addiction problem severity? *Alcohol Treat Q, 31*, 303–320.

Cano, I., Best, D., Edwards, M., & Lehman, J. (2017). Recovery capital pathways: Modelling the components of recovery wellbeing. *Drug and Alcohol Dependence, 181*, 11–19. https://doi.org/10.1016/j.drugalcdep.2017.09.002.

Center for Substance Abuse Treatment. (2005). *National Summit on Recovery Conference Report*. Paper presented at the National Summit on Recovery, Washington, D.C.

Chatterjee, S., Hovsepian, K., Sarker, H., Saleheen, N., Al'absi, M., Atluri, G., … Kumar, S. (2016). *mCrave: Continuous estimation of craving during smoking cessation*. In UbiComp'16 Proceedings of the 2016 ACM International Joint Conference on Pervasive and Ubiquitous Computing, pp. 863–874. https://doi.org/10.1145/2971648.2971672.

Ciciolla, L., Erato, G., Addante, S., Armans, M., & Quigley, A. (2020). Neonatal abstinence syndrome: caring for mothers and infants. In J. Croff & J. Beaman (Eds.), *Family resilience and recovery: Opioids and other addictions*. Springer. Manuscript submitted for publication.

Cleveland, H. H., & Harris, K. S. (2010). The role of coping in moderating within-day associations between negative triggers and substance use cravings: A daily diary investigation. *Addictive Behaviors, 35*(1), 60–63. https://doi.org/10.1016/j.addbeh.2009.08.010.

Cleveland, H. H., Harris, K. S., Baker, A. K., Herbert, R., & Dean, L. R. (2007). Characteristics of a collegiate recovery community: Maintaining recovery in an abstinence-hostile environment. *Journal of Substance Abuse Treatment, 33*, 13–23. https://doi.org/10.1016/j.jsat.2006.11.005.

Cleveland, H. H., Harris, K. S., & Wiebe, R. P. (Eds.). (2010). *Substance abuse recovery in college: Community supported abstinence* (Advancing responsible adolescent development). Springer. Retrieved from http://www.springer.com/series/7284

Dumont, F., & Vamos, P. (1975). The etiology and treatment of drug addiction: A problem in self concept and adaptation. *Addiction Therapist*.

Elliott, G., Kao, S., & Grant, A. (2004). Mattering: Empirical validation of a social-psychological concept. *Self and Identity, 3*(4), 339–354. https://doi.org/10.1080/13576500444000119.

Gómez, D., Jason, L. A., Contreras, R., DiGangi, J., & Ferrari, J. R. (2014). Vocational training and employment attainment among substance abuse recovering individuals within a communal living environment. *Therapeutic Communities, 35*(2), 42–47. https://doi.org/10.1108/TC-03-2014-0008.

Granfield, R., & Cloud, W. (1999). Coming clean: Overcoming addiction without treatment. New York: New York University Press.

Granfield, R., & Cloud, W. (2004). The Elephant that no one sees: Natural recovery among middle-class addicts. In J. Inciardi & K. McElrath (Eds.), The american drug scene: An anthology (4th ed.). Los Angeles, CA: H.W. Roxbury Publishing.

Groshkova, T., Best, D., & White, W. (2013). The assessment of recovery capital: Properties and psychometrics of a measure of addiction recovery strengths. *Drug and Alcohol Review, 32*, 187–194. https://doi.org/10.1111/j.1465-3362.2012.00489.x.

Harris, K.S., Baker, A.,, & Cleveland, H.H. (2010). Collegiate recovery communities: What they are and how they support recovery. In H.H. Cleveland, K.S. Harris, & R.P. Wiebe (Eds.), Substance abuse recovery in college: Community supported abstinence (pp. 9–22). Springer.

Hays-Grudo, J., Morris, A., Ratliff, E., & Croff, J. (2020). Adverse childhood experiences and addiction. In J. Croff & J. Beaman (Eds.), *Family resilience and recovery: Opioids and other addictions*. Springer. Manuscript submitted for publication.

Hennessy, E. A. (2017). Recovery capital: A systematic review of the literature. *Addiction Research & Theory, 25*(5), 349–360. https://doi.org/10.1080/16066359.2017.1297990.

Hovsepian, K., Al'Absi, M., Ertin, E., Kamarck, T., Nakajima, M., & Kumar, S. (2015). *cStress: Towards a gold standard for continuous stress assessment in the mobile environment.* UbiComp'15 – Proceedings of the 2015 ACM International Joint Conference on Pervasive and Ubiquitous Computing, 2015 (pp. 493–504). https://doi.org/10.1145/2750858.2807526.

Jason, L. A., & Ferrari, J. R. (2010). Oxford house recovery homes: Characteristics and effectiveness. *Psychological Services, 7*(2), 92–102. https://doi.org/10.1037/a0017932.

Jason, L. A., Olson, B. D., Ferrari, J. R., & Lo Sasso, A. T. (2006). Communal housing settings enhance substance abuse recovery. *American Journal of Public Health, 96*(10), 1727–1729. https://doi.org/10.2105/AJPH.2005.070839.

Kaskutas, L. A., Borkman, T. J., Laudet, A., Ritter, L. A., Witbrodt, J., Subbaraman, M. S., … Bond, J. (2014). Elements that define recovery: The experiential perspective. *Journal of Studies on Alcohol and Drugs, 75*, 999–1010. Retrieved from www.WhatIsRecovery.org

Kelly, J. F., & Hoeppner, B. (2015). A biaxial formulation of the recovery construct. *Addiction Research and Theory, 23*(1), 5–9. https://doi.org/10.3109/16066359.2014.930132.

Kelly, J. F., Bergman, B., Hoeppner, B. B., Vilsaint, C., & White, W. L. (2017). Prevalence and pathways of recovery from drug and alcohol problems in the United States population: Implications for practice, research, and policy. *Drug and Alcohol Dependence, 181*, 162–169. https://doi.org/10.1016/j.drugalcdep.2017.09.028.

Laudet, A. B. (2011). The case for considering quality of life in addiction research and clinical practice. *Addiction Science & Clinical Practice, 6*(1), 44–55. https://doi.org/10.1186/1940-0640-7-2.

Laudet, A. B., & Humphreys, K. (2013). Promoting recovery in an evolving policy context: What do we know and what do we need to know about recovery support services? *Journal of Substance Abuse Treatment, 45*, 126–133. https://doi.org/10.1016/j.jsat.2013.01.009.

Laudet, A. B., Harris, K., Kimball, T., Winters, K. C., & Moberg, D. P. (2015). Characteristics of students participating in collegiate recovery programs: A national survey. *Journal of Substance Abuse Treatment, 51*, 38–46. https://doi.org/10.1016/j.jsat.2014.11.004.

Molenaar, P. C. M. (2004). A manifesto on psychology as idiographic science: Bringing the person back into scientific psychology, this time forever. *Measurement, 2*(4), 201–218. https://doi.org/10.1207/s15366359mea0204_1.

Nesselroade, J. R., & Ram, N. (2004). Studying intraindividual variability: What we have learned that will help us understand lives in context. *Research in Human Development, 1*(1–2), 9–29. https://doi.org/10.1080/15427609.2004.9683328.

Olson, B., Jason, L. A., Davidson, M., & Ferrari, J. R. (2009). Increases in tolerance within naturalistic, intentional communities: A randomized, longitudinal examination. *American Journal of Community Psychology, 44*, 188–195. https://doi.org/10.1007/s10464-009-9275-3.

Oravecz, Z., & Brick, T. R. (2019). Associations between slow- and fast-timescale indicators of emotional functioning. *Social Psychological and Personality Science, 10*(7), 864-873. https://doi.org/10.1177/1948550618797128.

Osotsi, A., Oravecz, Z., Li, Q., Smyth, J., & Brick, T. R. (2020). Individualized modeling to distinguish between high and low arousal states using physiological data. *Journal of Healthcare Research Informatics*. https://doi.org/10.1007/s41666-019-00064-1.

Polcin, D. L., & Borkman, T. (2008). The impact of AA on non-professional substance abuse recovery programs and sober living houses. In M. Galanter, & L. Kaskutas (Eds.), *Recent Developments in Alcoholism, Vol 18: Alcoholics Anonymous and Spirituality in Addiction Recovery* (pp. 91–106). New York: Kluwer Academic/Plenum Publisher.

Polcin, D. L., Korcha, R. A., Bond, J., & Galloway, G. (2010). Sober living houses for alcohol and drug dependence: 18-month outcomes. *Journal of Substance Abuse Treatment, 38*, 356–365. https://doi.org/10.1016/j.jsat.2010.02.003.

Pritikin, J. N., Hunter, M. D., von Oertzen, T., Brick, T. R., & Boker, S. M. (2017). Many-level multilevel structural equation modeling: An efficient evaluation strategy. *Structural Equation*

Modeling: A Multidisciplinary Journal, 24(5), 684–698. https://doi.org/10.1080/10705511.2017.1293542.
Ram, N., & Diehl, M. (2015). *Multiple-time-scale design and analysis: Pushing toward real-time modeling of complex developmental processes.* In M. Diehl, K. Hooker, & M. J. Sliwinski (Eds.), *Handbook of intraindividual variability across the life span* (p. 308–323). Routledge/Taylor & Francis Group.
Russell, M., Cleveland, H. H., & Wiebe, R. P. (2010). Facilitating identity development in collegiate recovery: An Eriksonian perspective. In H.H. Cleveland, K.S. Harris, & R.P. Wiebe (Eds.), Substance abuse recovery in college: Community supported abstinence (pp. 23–35). Springer.
Smyth, J. M., Juth, V., Ma, J., & Sliwinski, M. (2017). A slice of life: Ecologically valid methods for research on social relationships and health across the life span. *Social and Personality Psychology Compass, 11*(10), 1–10. https://doi.org/10.1111/spc3.12356.
Snoke, J., Brick, T. R., Slavkovi, Ć. A., & Hunter, M. D. (2018). Providing accurate models across private partitioned data: Secure maximum likelihood estimation. *Annals of Applied Statistics, 12*(2), 877–914. https://doi.org/10.1214/18-AOAS1171.
Sobell, L. C., Ellingstad, T. P., & Sobell, M. B. (2000). Natural recovery from alcohol and drug problems: Methodological review of the research with suggestions for future directions. *Addiction, 95*(5), 749–764. Retrieved from https://search-proquest-com.ezaccess.libraries.psu.edu/docview/199685298/fulltextPDF/8348D40E32094B33PQ/1?accountid=13158
Sterling, R., Slusher, C., & Weinstein, S. (2008). Measuring recovery capital and determining its relationship to outcome in an alcohol dependent sample. *The American Journal of Drug and Alcohol Abuse, 34*, 603–610. https://doi.org/10.1080/00952990802308114.
Stone, A. A., & Shiffman, S. (1994). Ecological momentary assessment (EMA) in behavioral medicine. *Annals of Behavioral Medicine, 16*(3), 199–202.
Substance Abuse and Mental Health Services Administration (2011). *Results from the 2010 national survey on drug use and health: Summary of national findings, NSDUH Series H-41, HHS Publication No. (SMA) 11-4658.* Rockville, MD: Substance Abuse and Mental Health Services Administration
The Betty Ford Institute Consensus Panel. (2007). What is recovery? A working definition from the Betty Ford Institute. *Journal of Substance Abuse Treatment, 33*, 221–228.
Vilsaint, C. L., Kelly, J. F., Bergman, B. G., Groshkova, T., Best, D., & White, W. (2017). Development and validation of a Brief Assessment of Recovery Capital (BARC-10) for alcohol and drug use disorder. *Drug and Alcohol Dependence, 177*, 71–76. https://doi.org/10.1016/j.drugalcdep.2017.03.022.
White, W. L. (1998). *Slaying the dragon: The history of addiction treatment and recovery in America.* IL, USA: Chestnut Health Systems.
White, W. L. (2006). Recovery: The next frontier. In W. L. White, E. Kurtz, & M. Sanders (Eds.), *Recovery management* (pp. 1–6). Chicago: Great Lakes Addiction Technology Transfer Center (ATTC) Network.

Chapter 7
Seven Generations Mindset to Address Substance Use Disorders Among Native Americans

Rockey Robbins, R. Steven Harrist, and Bryan Stare

Colonial-settler violence has left a legacy of historical trauma with Native American people. Substance use has been one of the most destructive elements associated with the experience of historical trauma. Yet, Native Americans also have powerful healing legacies that can be utilized to restore tribal communities and their individual inhabitants to health. These legacies take the form of traditional healing practices, unique intergenerational and ecological relationships, values, and mindsets. This chapter offers information based on research, insights from critical Indigenous theory, and dialogue to gain insight about long-range foresight as a healthy guide to our behaviors. Of special interest to the authors of this chapter is the potential utility of cultivating an understanding of a mindset and consideration for the impact actions have on future generations.

1 Introduction: Seven Generations

The concept of "Seven Generations" is a principle that encourages people to make decisions in a way that considers the consequences of actions upon seven generations of people into the future. This idea of generational stewardship is believed to have first been documented in the Great Binding Law of the Iroquois (Welker 2016), which states "(1) look and listen for the welfare of the whole people and have always

R. Robbins (✉)
Jeannine Rainbolt College of Education, University of Oklahoma, Norman, OK, USA
e-mail: rockey@ou.edu

R. Steven Harrist
Oklahoma State University, Stillwater, OK, USA

B. Stare
University of North Carolina, Charlotte, OK, USA

J. M. Croff, J. Beaman (eds.), *Family Resilience and Recovery from Opioids and Other Addictions*, Emerging Issues in Family and Individual Resilience,
https://doi.org/10.1007/978-3-030-56958-7_7

in view not only the present but also the coming generations, even those whose faces are yet beneath the surface of the ground – the unborn of the future Nation." Although this does not explicitly reference several generations, the Haudenosaunee "Great Law of Peace" was originally an oral constitution, so the concept of "Seven Generations" has largely been passed down culturally (i.e., Cordova and Moore 2007; Lyons 1980). Indeed, though this concept has been frequently linked to environmental sustainability, it has also been echoed in modern discussions of organizational sustainability (Carleton 2009), community development (Jojola 2008), farming (Kruk-Buchowska 2018), education (Antone 2000; Looney 2011), and business (Tada 2012). This same precautionary concept is visibly present in current public discourse under the name intergenerational justice (Schuppert 2019; Smith 2019).

The phrase "Seven Generations" is commonly used in Indian Country today during conversations about combating substance use behaviors. The authors of this paper are fully aware that persons with substance use disorders have greater difficulties in delaying gratification for the "high" they desire or for the withdrawal they seek to avoid, and in their efforts to obtain their desired substance, they often do not demonstrate a concern about harming those with whom they are emotionally attached. The primary hypothesis of this chapter is that the "Seven Generations" mindset may contribute to preventative interventions and rehabilitation treatment provided by Native American behavioral health agencies. Individuals with substance use disorders live with great uncertainty and often struggle to maintain a healthy state and access necessities such as food, clothing, and shelter. This makes maintaining relationships with family and intimate partners, nurturing children, and cultivating intellectual curiosity difficult, and the conscious discrimination about one's impact on future generations is limited.

Despite the above limitations of the idea of "Seven Generations," our premise is that it may have potential usage in the fields of education and counseling. The primary limitation is that the complexities of the Seven Generations concept has been subjected to limited discussion, and therefore, until it has been comprehensively explored, it will be difficult to use it in educational and counseling contexts or research studies. This paper does not offer an exhaustive examination all the concept's latent meanings; however, it is a Chautauqua that begins a more profound consideration of this potentially powerful Native American concept. In the context of historical trauma, possibly the most discussed topic in Indian Country, combining the focus on history with future influences seems a natural fit. The written form of an oral dialogue is an attempt to both honor a long tradition of Native Americans coming together to engage in discourse on a topic and the spirit of Chautauqua.

2 Literature Review

Drug and alcohol addictions among Native Americans are associated with the experience of historical trauma, although to date there have been no studies correlating opioid use disorders and historical trauma among Native Americans. Over the past quarter century, the construct of historical trauma has become the pre-immanent focus in Native American psychological theories and research. The definition of historical trauma has shifted as decolonizing theorists and researchers have attempted to best utilize it in different contexts. In the early 1990s, Maria Yellow Horse Brave Heart, drawing from but differentiating the experiences of Holocaust survivors and Native Americans, described historical trauma as "historical legacies of colonization" (Brave Heart and DeBruyn 1998, p. 76). She wanted a conceptualization of historical trauma which would pre-empt "victim blaming and pathologizing" of Native Americans (Braveheart 1995, p. 8). Like other psychology researchers and theorists articulating the experience of Holocaust survivors, she believed that historical trauma was an unconscious transposition of the oppressed. However, she believed the previous focus on two-parent nuclear family systems was an erroneous perspective to be used with Native Americans. Consequently, she reconceptualized historical trauma in the context of Native American extended families in accordance with Native American community structures. Brave Heart (2003) defined historical trauma as "massive cumulative trauma across generations rather than the more limited diagnosis of ...Post Traumatic Syndrome Disorder, which is inadequate in capturing the influence and attributes of Native trauma" (pp. 7–8). She claimed that historical trauma impacts Native Americans with potential depressive symptoms, substance use disorders, fixation on trauma, and chronic pain.

There has also been an increased attempt to balance a psychological discourse about trauma with attention to socioeconomic, cultural, and structural factors (Gone 2014). Recent Native American critical scholars contextualize their works with settler-colonial theory which helps to delineate subtle and profound forms and arrangements of violence enacted upon Native Americans in past and present predicaments (Hartmann et al. 2019). They argue that the fields of education and psychology have often been guilty of pathologizing and stigmatizing Native American individuals because they have failed to consider the impact of the oppression they suffer under (Maxwell 2014).

Whitbeck has been in the forefront of creating space for research in establishing a relationship between historical trauma and substance use disorders. Whitbeck et al. (2004a, b) created the Historical Loss Scale (HLS) and the Historical Losses and Associated Symptoms Scale (HLASS), which expanded the focus on the effects of past colonialization to include contemporary oppressive experiences (Walls and Whitbeck 2012). Most studies over the last 15 years indicated a significant relationship between historical trauma and drug and alcohol addictions among Native Americans. In a study with 306 adult California Native Americans, Ehlers et al. (2013) found relationships between high HLS and HLASS scores and alcohol dependence. In a study with 459 Native American parents and caretakers, Whitbeck et al. (2004a, b) found that greater scores were associated with greater alcohol use disorders among women. And in a study of 120 urban Native American adults, Wiechelt et al. (2012) found that greater HLS scores were associated with more alcohol and illicit drug use. Researchers have continued illuminating a deeper understanding of the role of historical trauma in Native American addictions, providing a framework for destigmatizing conceptualization, and improving treatment practices (Breakout Box 7.1).

Breakout Box 7.1. Focus on Practice

As a trained clinical psychologist and a researcher, it is evident there is a need for more in-depth and exhaustive opioid research that is tailored to Tribal Nations to provide a better picture of opioid use among Native communities. The research is unclear and new research which guides clinical practice and shapes the medical culture is born out of the White community and is similar to mainstream culture because it starts in the doctor's office. The medical culture introduced opioids to Indian Country to manage pain. However, opioids are replaced with other methods as access is limited. Addiction is problematic among Native communities because of historical trauma, unresolved grief, and economic struggle, which calls for more refined studies that will inform clinical practice and challenge the disease model's focus on the individual. There is a specific need for community-wide interventions that use healing models built on culturally based empowerment and healing for Native communities to collectively recognize their resiliency, overcome historical trauma, and bring traditions back. Historical trauma is different so we need to do things differently clinically because standard in-patient care is not working. However, billing hinders clinicians from receiving reimbursement for community-based clinical services and funding is reserved specifically for individual level interventions. Native people do not trust mainstream clinical models to be confidential and safe. There is a warranted perception that if services are accessed everyone will know their business putting them at higher risk of losing their children, which highlights the need for referral systems with other tribes. Service delivery models must integrate a cultural assessment of the client to measure the constructs emphasized by the historical trauma model. Under this model, traditional Native people are allowed to grieve the losses of past generations free from the judgments rooted in the mainstream model that may wrongly deem this critical process as delusional and explore how their choices now carry forward in future generations. The models and ideas interwoven in clinical practice depend on the dynamic political climate, but seems to be open to a different way of thinking because the status quo remains ineffective in Indian country.

– Dr. Steven Ray Byers, Psychologist

White people have been increasingly impacted by the opioid epidemic, which has coincided with garnering ever-increasing public attention, but Native Americans have been more affected by the epidemic per capita than any other racial/ethnic group. On the surface, rates of all groups have been rising for 17 years with Native American rates seemingly comparable to those of Whites (Tipps et al. 2018), but this similarity may be grossly disproportionate upon closer examination (Joshi et al. 2018). For example, in Washington state from 2013 to 2015, Native Americans were more than 2.7 times more likely to die of an opioid-related overdose than Whites despite the two groups having similar opioid-related overdose death rates in the past

(Joshi et al. 2018). Researchers also found that Washington Native Americans were racially/ethnically misclassified on death certificates at a rate of 40% with such misclassification resulting in underestimation of opioid effects in Native American communities. These misclassifications and subsequent underestimations result in resource misallocations that leave Native American communities in further need of community-based prevention and treatment (Joshi et al. 2018). Statistics on opioid-related overdose deaths alone may also not accurately reflect the gravity of situations regionally in Native American communities either. It was hypothesized that the dire lack of available medical resources in certain tribal areas may preclude the availability and subsequent use of methamphetamine that appears to fill this void (Tipps et al. 2018). In other words, the severe lack of medical resources available to community members prevented opioid use disorders because they were unavailable even for medical necessity, but this trend was correlated with increased use of cheaper and more available methamphetamine.

In counter-distinction to the legacy of settler-colonial violence which brought about the historical trauma currently experienced by Native Americans, there is ongoing work toward wellness through the restoration of traditional Native American community health programs that encourage tribal healing practices. For example, the Elluam Tungiinun (wellness) cultural program in Alaska is an example of an Alaska Native/Native American community using tribal/cultural ideas and traditions to address substance use disorders and suicide (Rasmus 2014). They use Inuit words and concepts to explain the theoretical underpinnings of their healing approach. They explain that taking account of their Inuit geographic and cultural situation is crucial to healing their community. They carefully define key Inuit concepts that will guide what and how their work is conducted. Ellangneq means "becoming aware in one's growth into a real person." Elluam Tungiinun is defined as "toward wellness." Nunamta means "land and community." The program attempts to consider the interconnections between all in the community as well as their connections to the land and water. Yulgun means "peer influences," which remind all involved that healing does not always come from top down but involves young people as well as elders' wisdom. They have created tribally appropriate activities for their program participants, paying heed to ancient rituals and places. For instance, they conducted some of their healing, interactions around a qassgig, "dug-out fireplace," and in a boat on the cold ocean waters.

Some tribes are foregrounding traditional ideas and healing methods but supplement them with academic indigenous critical theories informed by writers such as and Brayboy (2006) and with Western psychological coping skills. Robbins et al. (2019) have been instrumental in combining tribal community ideas and ways with Western psychology in creating community psycho-educational groups and interventions to address substance use disorders. Among other traditional Native American healing techniques, they use smudging, Indian humor, sacred articles, stories, sweat baths, dances, and feasts to help individuals and communities move toward wellness. The challenge has been to ground these mixed approaches in each new community context. The guidance of elders in each tribal community has been critical.

The proceeding examples offer traces of the wisdom that should be considered for passing down to future generations. As stated in the introduction, the primarily cognitive mindset of "Seven Generations" is not enough to transform the lives of most people experiencing addiction to drugs and alcohol. Still, as has been argued, a "Seven Generations" mindset may offer a mental approach and framework to guide us into the future.

3 Seven Generations/Legacy

The following dialogue is an attempt to help readers understand the profundity and complexity of the idea of "Seven Generations." Steve Harrist and I had initially planned to create psycho-educational group activities based on the concept of legacy. The groups would have consisted of Native American adolescents and their parents. However, we decided it was necessary to first engage in several "intense" discussions about the definition of legacy and "Seven Generations." I kept notes as we talked. Steve died before the notes could be translated into psycho-educational activities as planned. What follows are thought fragments, personal asides, and sometimes exact quotations that were joined to create the following dialogue. I hope they are valuable in contributing to an understanding of legacy and/or "Seven Generations." Steve argued that trainings of any kind without deep understanding of the issues would inevitably lack substance and dynamism. It is our sincere desire that the following discussion provides the basis for a profound understanding of the "Seven Generations" idea.

3.1 Dialogue

Rockey (R): Talking about substance abuse among Native Americans in a tribal/cultural context must be preliminary to trying to address it in tribal communities because without a tribally appropriate understanding, interventions are bound to result in as many problems as they might solve.

Steve (S): What are some of the views that Natives have about the abuse of "drugs?"

R: Medicine people are hesitant about providing potions or herbs. The medicine people I have worked with believe that we should let nature take its course and we should be patient. Then if medicine is needed, it should be used with respect. When persons in my family and I myself have worked with medicine people, medicine is typically used within the context of ritual. There is singing and often water and/or heat. They have told me that hard drugs without ritual and moderation wreak havoc. I once heard an elder road man or peyote meeting leader give a long "lecture" to a young man who was suspected of using peyote outside of ritual.

S: So, the peyote meeting leader was attempting to pass down wisdom about medicines to this person of a younger generation. Legacy is typically associated with passing on money or property to children and grandchildren, but knowledge and wisdom may be even a more valuable legacy.

R: Yes, many tribal people use the phrase, "Seven Generations," which is about behaving in such a way that you think about how your choices and actions will impact the world in seven generations.

S: Too often people think of the material things that can be passed on which is in line with contemporary focuses on empirical reality, but interior introspection and feelings can be let go into the world to impact people for generations to come. Sadly, even our educational field is unappreciative of these more meditative and internal traditions, with its heavy emphasis on empirical knowledge.

R: I think that Native Americans possess great wisdoms that would be helpful in combating addictions. Helping people to look at their interior worlds could aid in immunizing persons against drug and alcohol abuse. I think promoting this mindset of "Seven Generations" could be a key element.

S: Having a long-range view of our influence is to see ourselves beyond our finite, time-limited existences. I believe we are more than an encapsulated self within a body. How does this look specifically for Native Americans?

R: We regularly talk about spiritual experiences in which we have realized that we are part of everything. I don't think it is necessary to engage in traditional Native ceremonies to experience this, but I think participation in sweats, peyote meetings, traditional dances, and other ceremonies can help to elicit these experiences. Combining these experiences with traditional teaching about healthy living and a mindfulness about our responsibilities to future generations can aid people who struggle with addiction. Many Native Americans would do well to go back and find the good in these traditional ways and values. They are powerful legacies.

S: Passing down these bodies of knowledge about healthy living, which have been accumulated over centuries, may have been interrupted by colonialization. I am glad some people have kept them. When we were in the sweat lodge, listening to the stories and the traditional chants, I began reflecting on some profound issues. We are going to die. Even if we live 100 years, and I may die a lot earlier, the life sequence on earth goes on. The old tree dies, but an acorn from that tree, if it is nurtured, grows into the future and bears its fruit. Having this mindset, if it is taken to heart, may help to immunize people from drug and alcohol abuse.

R: Yes, unitary experiences elicited in ceremonies help us to realize the shared energy we have with those who came before us and those who will come after us. It is important for us to honor those who came before us and those who follow us.

S: Are you saying that a part of appreciating the concept of legacy is feeling a responsibility or even an obligation for people of future ages? That bothers me a little bit. I don't want anyone feeling responsible for honoring my life by the way they live. That would alienate that person from living their own life. We cannot live for those who come before us. I used to think I had to achieve full professorship because my father had not attained that. Was that really honoring him? Do I want my kids to lead lives to honor me? No. Each generation faces their own unique challenges. As parents we hope we can offer nurturance and some good, but they deserve to have freedom to become who they are in a way that is unbridled by trying to honor us. They honor us by exploring who they are within their unique circumstances.

R: Point well taken. I can see how an element of obligation could be guilt provoking and restricting. Our time individually is a time of growth that can go in many directions. There may be a little difference in this regard for Native Americans as we have been more collectivist. Our legacy has been one of death and destruction. If we give up our ways completely, we lose what is valuable for our people. I do feel some responsibility to practice our old ways. Our elders often speak of being worthy of what has brought us this far. The old Tsalagi ways, ka no he lv hi, must be preserved or we lose our unique identities.

S: No, I see your point. Individuals in collectivist societies may find their worth in working to create future possibilities that they themselves cannot partake in in their present conditions.

R: Yes, but I think that sounds more like a Marxist perspective. We probably think a little more in terms of preserving our traditions which are embedded in the past but have the potential for contributing to the continued existence of our people. Yes, and I think our idea of the preservation of traditions are an element of collectivist ideology.

S: But such a collectivist perspective does not necessarily negate individual expression. Those sacred tree roots of ancestors are in each of us and in some sense the future tree is in us too, but each individual life is ours to enjoy. As individuals we may have to sift through all the crud to see what is of worth. We may have to make difficult choices as individuals to discover those connections you mention.

R: It is those connections that are important to emphasize if we are to maintain our unique tribal identities, while at the same time encouraging unique actualizations related to our own uniquenesses. Everything changes, but we think some things are worth preserving.

S: Nothing in this world is ever really lost. It is all connected. The future absorbs what has come before it, which is why living healthy lives promotes health in the future. This notion of the present and future absorbing the past is relevant to our concept of legacy.

R: I think for Native Americans this question has unique aspects. Writers like Toynbee and Spengler wrote about the rise and decline of cultural traditions, some just decaying while others were destroyed. With Native Americans, traditions did not decay and disappear, rather colonists purposely tried to annihilate them. For many tribes, only a little cultural capital has survived and less truly reclaimed.

S: I see what you mean. I think for many White people, there is the notion that legacy contributes to the ongoing progress of humankind. But your example demonstrates this comes from a White-centric, even an American-centric positioning. The historical trauma that Native Americans suffer from today is the result of actions taken by White people who were and are convinced that their ways are an integral part of Manifest Destiny. But everything is not necessarily culminating into a Utopia and lots are being lost that was very good. Today technology is assumed by some to be what will save us, bring about a world of peace, but with all its positives it is also more lethal than ever and can be used for evil, tyrannical reasons.

R: Yes. One of the most colonizing ideas is that we are living in a world that is gradually maturing toward a fulfillment.

S: I have thought a lot about this. We may want to leave a "good" legacy, but the ultimate outcomes of our actions are obscure. We can never know what we transfer to future generations no matter how we consciously direct our actions.

R: The opioid crisis is a perfect example of this. Modern medicine is viewed as an advancement, but it too is often used in destructive ways and not just by people suffering from addiction. The medical establishment is sometimes motivated by greed and favors White folks more than people of color.

S: But again, what specifically is it that has been lost in Native American cultures that might help promote health among Native Americans?

R: I think we must do a lot of decolonizing before we can really get at this regarding drug and alcohol abuse. I was discussing this topic with some Native American friends the other day and they said that they saw drug and alcohol addicts as heroic in their struggle against being subsumed by White colonization. I think this is a powerful thought, worthy of serious discussion.

S: Only an ignorant or close-minded person could fail to see the source of the destructive behavior of drug and alcohol abuse in the cruel efforts of White dominant society's attempt to annihilate Native American cultures.

R: We are not viewed as human beings in our own right. We are only perceived as human if we abandon our cultural identities and fit into the overwhelming White education, political, health, and religious systems. Some Native Americans believe it would be better to destroy themselves by abusing substances than to lose themselves in the White system.

S: I am positioned in such a way, as a White person with maybe some Native heritage, that I am having a difficult time responding to these remarks. Any remark I might make to try to inspire hope is to climb up on a hill to make a hypocritical moral pronouncement. I totally see why Native Americans might rather destroy themselves than to fit into a system that does not respect their unique ontologies. I cognitively know the history of genocide against Native Americans but can't possibly understand it on a visceral level.

R: I appreciate you. It is this humility and lack of defensiveness that allows for a real discussion. You see, I think there are some elements of self-deception in the pessimistic reasoning I have mentioned, but we do not need White people telling us about it. Drug and alcohol abuse might be a rationalization at times for a loss of connection and hope. First, one must consider the suffering of family members that accompanies such an unconscious or conscious choice to put one's vitality at risk with drug and alcohol abuse. Secondly, I think our traditions have historically considered a vertical connection no matter how incredibly oppressive any situation is. This allows for freedom that White hegemony can never obscure or destroy.

S: Let me be clear. Are you saying the resisting attitude and opinion you expressed about using drugs and alcohol against White hegemony might at times evolve into despair? And it might lead to loneliness and believing you have nothing to live for?

R: First let me reiterate the critical, even pessimistic view, in response to the attempted genocide. Without a highly critical perspective and active resistance, we not only remain in ignorance, we are also robbed of the will to overcome injustices. But on the other hand, I think this cynical view has the potential to shift all responsibility and blame for the problems we face in our lives and our tribe's continuance upon others. We cannot ignore that we have some cultural capital at our disposal that we can tap into, and we have a long history of being a spiritual people whose vertical connection to our Creator has transcended our oppressive predicaments. While a pessimistic perspective gives us a critical perspective, on the emotional level it might lead to despair and destructive life styles.

S: I would add that fear is also an elemental pathway to all kinds of destruction. It comes in many guises and may evolve into despair. We are deeply afraid of death, and we are afraid of life. We fear we have wasted our lives, for instance, by the abuse of drugs and alcohol. But we are afraid of looking deep within for the power to change because we are not sure what else we might find there. We may have to look back at things we have done that we can no longer change. But if we would only go there, we would find we can gain inner knowledge, power, and peace.

R: It is not too late for a person who is abusing substances to begin again with a new standard of values. Native Americans have had hundreds of years of trial, but we are still here. Of course, it takes a firm decision and a dedication to change, but it is possible. Look at nature. It renews itself continually. Life is always changing and there is little that cannot be made better. I would add that a visionary perspective or what Cherokees call "ago us do di" is invaluable. It is to be open to help and healing from unlikely sources, even from a spiritual reality invisible to the eyes. It is also to see opportunity in challenging situations. It is not scientific but is a choice to live within our circles of tribal religious faith.

S: You mention the vertical connection. Alcoholics Anonymous teaches that in order to free ourselves from the miserable and unhappy predicament the abuse of drugs and alcohol situates us in, it is necessary to remold our spirit to the will of God.

R: Some Native Americans would argue that vertical, which I have used, is not the right word because it is God's imminence that is more emphasized in Native American religions, but while this is true, the transcendent element of God is also emphasized in most tribes. I was told by a Native elder that the medicine people looked for many centuries for the source of life in their deep meditations and finally concurred that there is an invisible creative force from which all life springs. The Creator is in some sense apart from its creation as well as a part of it. But I guess the point is that a connection to this Creative Source results in a deep belief that despite the apparent threat of the ultimate genocide of Native American cultures, the good will eventually win.

S: And that may be associated with a desire to at least try to live a healthy life. I think it is vital to make a commitment to live as though nothing is ever set in stone. As we work on or try to work on just living in a healthy way, things may change. You know, never give in to the challenges of living; something may be at work in our lives that could change everything. I can hope for more life here, but if I don't get it, something lives on, hopefully for the good.

R: Having faith in something beyond us that knows a lot of variables that we may not know, is reasonable to me. We use the phrase "di gu go ta nv" to describe the use of good judgment. We do best to choose what our conscience tells us even when we are moving through situations that are troublesome and even when we are not treated fairly by dominant powers in society.

S: I am reminded of a story I read about a woman who was confined behind bars in a Nazi concentration camp. She was beaten and tortured but continued to be kind to her torturer. The freedom we always have is to love despite how we are treated, and this may be participating in a destiny larger than we understand.

R: I respect her capacity to love and experience moments of joy despite horrendous oppression. There is a legacy of love that we may participate in which may insolate us from drug and alcohol abuse.

S: As you know, hermeneutics philosophy has been a passion of mine. It primarily has to do with understanding each other so that we can escape our isolated egos into understanding ourselves as "we" rather than "I." It is about working toward a mutual feeling of resonance. It can only start from this kind of honest uncomfortable dialogue we are having now. I want to add that love must have justice as bones, else it is flimsy. We also live in situations that we might not choose, yet within that prison we have some freedom in how we experience it.

R: I am confronted with what is my generation going to leave behind even as I consider the current inequities and racism we experience in this White system? I don't want mine to be leaving behind an influence on our children that will contribute to the continued abuse of alcohol and drugs.

S: Before continuing this conversation about legacy, I think it is important to remind our egos that we cannot really predict the lasting influence we might have on the world that follows our existence. The ultimate end of my actions is obscure to me. No matter how intentional my actions, I cannot guess their final influence. Our egos become inflated if we inflate the importance our individual legacies.

R: Good point. Shelly's "Ozymandias" reminds us that even the most powerful emperor's legacies turn to dust. Teotitlan in Mexico City is nothing but rubble. Yet, on the other hand, our elders never cease to remind us that the dust of our ancestors in the ground beneath our feet is sacred.

S: Yes. It is a good thing to provide our children with what they need to make them spiritually strong and capable of understanding the importance of acting in a way that is thoughtful for others.

R: The Cherokee word for gift is adahnehdi. We might at least help to set the next generations free to be caretakers of the earth. I have been taught by my elders that nothing is ever lost. The old ones seem to disappear like the morning midst when the sun comes out. They are gone it seems, but….

S: Yes, yes. Nothing may ever be really lost. And being in time and space may enhance what is dear to us. We may look back and think someone no longer exists. But making a meal with your wife while listening to the joyful bantering of your son and daughter may not just be a forgotten moment but may live forever.

R: Humor and genuine love may persist, may renew itself in the next generation as well as continuing in some sense on an eternal plane.

S: Love is what really ends up mattering. Everything that appears on earth disappears. The meaning of most everything is ultimately hidden from us. We turn the page, and everything appears to be gone. Death appears to destroy everything. I cannot prove it, but I feel it and I think I hear inner voices that tell me that something continues in the beyond and some part of us continues this earth.

R: I think it is hard to hear those reassuring voices clearly when we are addicted to drugs and alcohol. Without what we call to hi dv or inner peace, it is hard to develop our spirits. Leaving a positive legacy requires the development of our inner spirits …. But I can get cynical sometimes, especially when there is too much talk about hope and love. I mean look at how the cycles of destruction keep repeating themselves. I believe human beings have some freedom to change, but there is something about our species that seems to be destructive to others and to ourselves.

S: I believe we can break the destructive cycles with our freedom to make good choices. We may not see the end of our efforts to make the world a better place or predict what it will be, but we can live in such a way that may contribute to a new and better world. I believe our persistence to make a better world can make a difference. But we cannot be short-term thinkers and workers. We must persist. It may take generations, but we can contribute to positive change.

R: For generations many Native Americans have had little choice but to struggle to survive. Not all but many. To think about our people accomplishing a tribally focused good is difficult for many of us. So much of our unique cultural capital has been stripped from us that when we try to articulate what a better new world would be like, the words come out like a White person is saying them. I want our goals to be articulated in our tribal languages.

S: Purpose should be more than making selfish intentional goals. Everything we have talked about suggests that historically Native Americans have thought more in terms of extended family and tribal terms than individualistic ones. So, the point of freeing oneself from addictions must be set in the context of its effects upon those around them and upon future generations.

R: But I think as you have stated earlier, there is also a subjective meaning. Again, in Cherokee we say, di gu go t nv or good judgment. Each of us must make good judgments bring about positive changes. Yes, our tribal communities' futures are important, but tribes are made up of individuals. We should not go too far with the idea that Native Americans think only in collectivistic terms.

S: Legacy starts with knowing your worth, loving yourself. You really can't even feel that you have purpose unless you can appreciate the life you have been given. Then you can know deep down that there is something worth passing on. You can then see yourself as a contributing part of a community.

R: Death is also a crucial part the process of legacy. We have a localized self in time and space that influences the world we live in and then we die. It comes back to what, if any, individual responsibility do we have?

S: Maybe to teach our children to watch a wave come all the way into shore or to hold their breath to hear a song of a bird or a chord on a guitar or the voice in a vocal performance. Maybe we are here to learn to appreciate and love everything and pass that on. Could it be that simple sometimes?

R: As individuals I recollect back into circular Nature, maybe even into God, but I leave a trace behind, though I can never be sure about its effect. Does this help in meeting death bravely? I know that a lot of peoples' lives are just about surviving or accumulating transitory material assists. But I do think some people want to feel they have a larger purpose. Believing that our lives may have a chance to positively impact our tribal people in the future, the species in general, is a powerful purpose. It entails thinking about the consequences of our behavior for the world in seven generations. I think when people have purpose, long-range purpose, it can change the way they live.

S: For me, believing that my love mattered for those who go forward with mortal life is meaningful. The positive legacy I want is to help people move to a new state of growth in the directions they can be happy even if it is without me.

R: I think people who are near death may be more likely to think about what their lives count for in the long run. But when our elders talked about behaving in a way to impact the world in seven generations, they wanted people even in the prime of their lives to have such a mindset.

3.2 Summary of Main Themes of Dialogue

We discussed the concept of Seven Generations as a mindset in contra-distinction to the symptoms of feelings of hopelessness, fear, and worthlessness, which are symptoms of historical trauma. Unique Native American values, attitudes, beliefs, concepts, rituals, and ways of communicating were spoken of as vital legacies to maintain and restore health to tribal individuals and communities. We complicated any idealistic notion of Seven Generations by noting that we never know what the lasting effects of our living traces might be because of ever-shifting historical circumstances. Further, even the most seemingly positive aspects of our lives have the potential of dictating our descendants' lives in such a way that their unique gifts might be dampened if adhered to too closely. Ultimately, we can only hope to live lives that promote some sort of goodness through the love we share and the healthy choices we make and by honoring our unique tribal ways. We reflected about the impacts that maniacal genocidal attacks upon Native Americans as well as current structurally oppressive relationships with societal structures characterized by systemic racism. We considered the potential benefits of the collectivist traditional tribal values such as beliefs in vertical spiritual connections that transcend time and space, the interdependence of all living things, and interconnections with future descendants. We discussed the potential benefits of foresight mindsets for individuals and communities.

4 Discussion

In the past, there have been small groups who attempted to introduce a new width of intellectuality to their time. They may not have seen their ideas come to fruition, yet decades, centuries, or even thousands of years later their thought manifested in action (Whitehead 1933). For decades, ecologists have challenged us to think about how our behavior may result in the destruction of earth if we did not change. Today, we are already seeing the results of our callous disregard for future generations in climate change and rising water levels (Schuppert 2019). In general, our individual behaviors and our community planning are largely dominated by businesses which have been infected by the disease of short-sightedness (Colbert 2020). Too often, as individuals may think in terms of immediate needs or we may be locked into thinking about our immediate needs or desires.

This paper is an argument for a general philosophic foresight outlook to guide our actions to influence the future in a positive way. We focused our foresight outlook in relation to drug and alcohol problems that are destroying an inordinate number of lives, especially in Native American communities (Ehlers et al. 2013). Foregrounding tribal values are paramount. We advocate a general education that would convey a philosophic outlook of noble sentiments for the future that entails tribal virtues of reverence, courage, and vision. The Cherokee ideas of respecting ka no he lv hi ("old ways"), making di gu go ta nv ("good judgments") and having ago us do di ("vision or openness to opportunities or positive outlook"), are key elements in primary elements in a Seven Generations mentality. The dialogue portion of this paper begins the educative aspect of this work as it is an attempt to promote understanding of the complexity of this mindset of foresight. Trainings would include the use of current psychological and physiological phraseology to activate participants to internalize ideas regarding foresight. It is our hope that the above research and dialogue about the concept of Seven Generations may contribute to efforts to build healing models to address tribal experiences of historical trauma and substance abuse.

Glossary of Terms

Colonialism the act or policy of a country seeking to extend or retain its authority over other people or territories, generally with the aim of economic dominance

Historical trauma trauma that spans experienced by a specific cultural, racial, or ethnic group multiple generations

Racism prejudice or discrimination against a person or people on the basis of their racial or ethnic group

Questions for Thought and Discussion

1. How do you think how your choices will impact the world in the future? Has this changed your behavior?
2. How do you envision using the concept of "Seven Generations" to address tribal experiences of historical trauma and substance abuse? How could it be used to help other racial groups with historical trauma and substance abuse?
3. What do you want your legacy to be?
4. If you have been affected by historical trauma, how has this manifested in your life? If not, what do you see your role is to help those process their historical trauma?

References

Antone, E. M. (2000). Empowering aboriginal voice in aboriginal education. *Canadian Journal of Native Education, 24*(2), 92–101. Retrieved from https://search-proquest-com.ezproxy.lib.ou.edu/docview/230307757?accountid=12964

Braveheart, M. Y. H. (1995). *The return to the sacred path: Healing from historical trauma and historical unresolved grief among the Lakota* (Doctoral dissertation). Smith College School for Social Work.

Braveheart, M. Y. H. (2003). The historical trauma response among natives and its relationship with substance abuse: A Lakota illustration. *Journal of Psychoactive Drugs, 35*, 7–13. https://doi.org/10.1080/02791072.2003.10399988.

Braveheart, M. Y. H., & DeBruyn, L. M. (1998). The American Indian holocaust: Healing historical unresolved grief. *American Indian and Alaska Native Mental Health Research, 8*, 56–78. https://doi.org/10.5820/aian.0802.1998.60.

Brayboy, B. M. J. (2006). Toward a tribal critical race theory in education. *The Urban Review, 37*(5), 425–446. https://doi.org/10.1007/s11256-005-0018-y.

Carleton, K. L. (2009). Framing sustainable performance with the Six-P. *Performance Improvement, 48*(8), 37–44. https://doi.org/10.1002/pfi.20101.

Colbert, E. (2020). *The case for catastrophe.* Washington, DC: National Geographic, National Geographic Partners. ISSN 0027-9358.

Cordova, V. F., & Moore, K. D. (2007). *How it is: The native American philosophy of V.F. Cordova.* Tucson: University of Arizona Press.

Ehlers, C. L., Gizer, I. R., Gilder, D. A., Ellingson, J. M., & Yehuda, R. (2013). Measuring historical trauma in an American Indian community sample: Contributions of substance dependence, affective disorder, conduct disorder, and PTSD. *Drug and Alcohol Dependence, 133*, 180–187. https://doi.org/10.1016/j.drugrugalcdep.2013.05.011.

Gone, J. P. (2014). Reconsidering American Indian historical trauma: Lessons from an early Gros ventre war narrative. *Transcultural Psychiatry, 51*, 387–406. https://doi.org/10.1177/1363461513489722.

Hartmann, W. E., Wendt, D. C., Burrage, R. L., Palmerville, A., & Gone, J. P. (2019). American Indian historical trauma: Anti-colonial prescriptions for healing, resilience, and survivance. *American Psychologist, 74*(1), 6–19. https://doi.org/10.1037/amp0000326.

Jojola, T. (2008). Indigenous planning: An emerging context. *Canadian Journal of Urban Research, 17*(1), 37–47. Retrieved from https://search-proquest-com.ezproxy.lib.ou.edu/docview/208739515?accountid=12964

Joshi, S., Weiser, T., & Warren-Mears, V. (2018). *Drug opioid-involved, and heroin-involved overdose deaths among American Indians and Alaska Natives – Washington, 1999–2015*. MMWR. https://doi.org/10.15585/mmwr.mm6750a2.

Kruk-Buchowska, Z. (2018). Transnationalism as a decolonizing strategy? 'Trans-indigenism' and native American food sovereignty. *Studia Anglica Posnaniensia, 53*(1), 413–423. https://doi.org/10.2478/stap-2018-0020.

Looney, P. B. (2011). President's letter. *Environmental Practice, 13*(2), 81–82. https://doi.org/10.1017/S1466046611000159.

Lyons, O. (1980). The Iroquois tree of peace. In C. Vecsey & R. W. Venables (Eds.), *American Indian environments: Ecological issues in native American history* (pp. 173–174). Syracuse: Syracuse University Press.

Maxwell, K. (2014). Historicizing historical *trauma* theory: Troubling the transgenerational transmission paradigm. *Transcultural Psychiatry, 51*, 407–435. https://doi.org/10.1177/1363461514531317.

Rasmus, S. M. (2014). Indigenizing CBPR: Evaluation of a community-based and participatory research process implementation of the Elluam Tungiinun (towards wellness) program in Alaska. *American Journal of Community Psychology, 54*, 170–179. https://doi.org/10.1007/s10464-014-9653-3.

Robbins, R. R., Stare, B. G., & Riggins, B. R. (2019). Through the Diamond Threshold: A community-based psycho-educational group training program for treatment of substance use disorders among American Indians. *American Indian and Alaska Native Mental Health Research, 26*(1), 79–105. https://doi.org/10.5820/aian.2601.2019.79.

Schuppert, F. (2019). *Climate change and intergenerational justice*. Unicef. Retrieved from https://www.unicef-irc.org/article/920-climate-change-and-intergenerational-justice.html

Smith, S. (2019). Pete Buttigieg wants 'intergenerational justice.' What's that? *NBC News*. Retrieved from https://www.nbcnews.com/politics/2020-election/pete-buttigieg-wants-intergenerational-justice-what-s-n978316

Tada, K. (2012). Social behaviors in first nations businesses: An exploration of alternative development. *The Canadian Journal of Native Studies, 32*(2), 77–101. Retrieved from https://search-proquest-com.ezproxy.lib.ou.edu/docview/1498365291?accountid=12964

Tipps, R. T., Buzzard, G. T., & McDougall, J. A. (2018). The opioid epidemic in Indian country. *The Journal of Law, Medicine & Ethics, 46*, 422–443. https://doi.org/10.1177/1073110518782950.

Walls, M. L., & Whitbeck, L. B. (2012). Advantages of stress process approaches for measuring historical trauma. *The American Journal of Drug and Alcohol Abuse, 38*, 416–420. https://doi.org/10.3109/00952990.2012.694524.

Welker, G. (2016). *Constitution of the Iroquois Nations*. Retrieved from http://www.indigenouspeople.net/iroqcon.htm

Whitbeck, L. B., Adams, G. W., Hoyt, D. R., & Chen, X. (2004a). Conceptualizing and measuring historical trauma among American Indian people. *American Journal of Community Psychology, 33*, 119–130. https://doi.org/10.1023/B:AJCP.0000027000.777357.31.

Whitbeck, L. B., Chen, X., Hoyt, D. R., & Adams, G. W. (2004b). Discrimination, historical loss, enculturation: Culturally specific risk and resiliency factors for alcohol abuse among American Indians. *Journal of Studies on Alcohol, 65*, 409–418. https://doi.org/10.15288/jsa.2004.65.409.

Whitehead, A. N. (1933). *Adventures of the mind*. New York: Macmillan.

Wiechelt, S., Gryczynski, J., Johnson, J., & Caldwell, D. (2012). Historical trauma among American Indians: Impact on substance abuse and family cohesion. *Journal of Loss and Trauma, 17*, 319–336. https://doi.org/10.1080/15325024.2011.616837.

Chapter 8
Associations Between SUD in the Family, PFC Functioning, and Codependency: Importance of Family Member Recovery

Spencer D. Bradshaw, Sterling T. Shumway, and Thomas G. Kimball

1 Introduction

Family units play a profound role in the development of individual behavior, health, and well-being. From a family systems theoretical perspective, individuals' thinking, feelings, and behavior influence the family "atmosphere," and the family atmosphere reciprocally influences each individual's thinking, feelings, and behavior (Kerr et al. 1988). Therefore, individual illness and well-being impact the whole (i.e., the family), and the family impacts the individuals of which it is comprised. It is from this perspective that the understanding of substance use disorders (SUDs) as a "family disease" has emerged (Roth 2010).

Similar to other chronic illnesses, if one family member experiences an illness (e.g., a substance use disorder), each family member is impacted (Rolland 1993), despite the family member with a diagnosed illness is identified as the "patient" (Schwartz and Nichols 2004). As a family system organizes itself to respond to the loved one with an SUD, family functioning is negatively impacted (Moos and Moos 1984) and may result in broken marriages and parent-child relationships, abuse, and other physical and mental health illnesses (Schäfer 2011). As an emotional unit, the family atmosphere may emphasize stress and emotional pain associated with decreased health and functioning of each family member. Research has shown that family members of those with an SUD are more likely to be diagnosed with depression or with their own substance use disorder (Ray et al. 2007), and that these family members in

S. D. Bradshaw (✉)
Human Development and Family Studies Department, Utah State University, Logan, UT, USA
e-mail: spencer.bradshaw@usu.edu

S. T. Shumway · T. G. Kimball
Texas Tech University, Lubbock, TX, USA
e-mail: sterling.shumway@ttu.edu; thomas.kimball@ttu.edu

J. M. Croff, J. Beaman (eds.), *Family Resilience and Recovery from Opioids and Other Addictions*, Emerging Issues in Family and Individual Resilience,
https://doi.org/10.1007/978-3-030-56958-7_8

general have higher medical costs and claims (Ray et al. 2007; Weisner et al. 2010). Of critical importance, medical claims are also higher when family members do not have direct involvement in their loved one's SUD treatment (Spear and Mason 1991).

Unfortunately, family members of those with an SUD are often neglected, do not have the resources or support needed for their own health (Orford et al. 2010, 2013), and could develop a "codependency." Codependency has a history of being difficult to define, however, research has shown that it has four "core features," including (1) an excessive external focus on or concern regarding others, (2) "self-sacrificing" behaviors or putting others needs before one's own, (3) attempts to control, and (4) difficulty experiencing and expressing emotions (Dear et al. 2005). Codependency is typically considered a "learned" condition (Chang 2012) that results in "enabling" behaviors, which when left unchanged may sustain continued use for the person with the SUD. Therefore, involving family members in treatment has often emphasized skills and tools for reduction of enabling behaviors in order to enhance ability to support recovery for their loved one. While family is an important support system for SUD recovery (England Kennedy and Horton 2011), it is equally important to focus on the well-being and recovery of family members themselves, in addition to recovery for their loved one (Shumway et al. 2019).

Additional research on the impact SUDs have on a family system is needed to bring more focus, resources, and care toward family members. Specifically, research is needed that may further identify the impact of SUDs on the health and well-being of family members. For example, given the stressful environment associated with decreased family functioning, and associations between stress, brain functioning, and disease (McEwen 2012), it is likely that family members experience neurological impacts that associate with enabling behaviors and reduced personal health. Research showing that family members are impacted at a neurological level would provide understanding that their experiences and responses within an SUD context are not solely based on personal preferences and decisions (much like a person with an SUD does not continue use solely due to a lack of moral decision-making). Additionally, there may be greater recognition of the importance of recovery of each individual family member, and of the family as a whole. Additionally, and in systemic fashion, as each family member finds health and recovery, families, collectively, can become healthier atmospheres and more effective support systems to those with SUDs.

1.1 Addiction as a Family Disease

As previously mentioned, a family systems perspective emphasizes that the family is an emotional unit that both influences and is influenced by individual family member thoughts, feelings, and behaviors (Kerr et al. 1988). This mutual influence arises out of the Aristotelian view that "the whole is more than the sum of its parts" (Von Bertalanffy 1972, p. 407). Failing to recognize the reciprocal influence between the thoughts, feelings, and behaviors of each family member and the family atmosphere—and instead focusing on only one side of this mutual interaction—is like "forgetting that mass depends on gravity as much as gravity depends on mass" (Kerr et al. 1988). This holistic view of the family increases understanding of SUDs as a family disease, which involves the family unit and relationships organizing themselves toward a homeostasis centered around the substance use (Steinglass 1985). This homeostasis is maintained by shifts of important family dynamics—including family power dynamics, rules, roles, and boundaries; all of which ultimately shape family structure.

1.1.1 Family Power Dynamics

Power can be defined as the relative influence that each family member has on the course or outcome of an activity. Power often, therefore, occurs in a hierarchy and is associated with how families demand, protect, reward, punish, and shape interactions of family members (Broderick 1993; Broderick and Smith n.d.). Various factors may be involved regarding who in a family holds the most power (Broderick 1993). However, from a Western worldview, in families where a SUD is present, it is often the SUD itself that holds the majority of power (Krestan 2000). Interestingly, this perspective is likely associated with the first step and premise of 12-step recovery approaches (Reiter 2014), in which one acknowledges *powerlessness* over their problematic substance use and that life has become unmanageable (Alcoholics Anonymous 2001). From an Al-anon 12-step perspective for family members impacted by an SUD, family members also acknowledge powerlessness over their loved one and their problematic substance use (How Al-Anon Works for Families and Friends of Alcoholics 1995). One way the allocation of power to the SUD in the family system manifests is through family rules that often fail to promote change and recovery from the SUD.

1.1.2 Family Rules

Family systems are in part governed by rules that regulate individuals' behavior and also influence their thoughts and feelings. Ideally, family rules would be fair and flexible (Black 2002) and would benefit each family member by promoting health and growth. However, like power, rules also shift over time in ways that close the family off from important resources and conversations and, therefore, may support continued substance use or hinder recovery. According to Black (2002), three common rules that have been identified in families in the midst of struggles with an SUD and result in the family becoming a closed system are *don't talk, don't trust,* and *don't feel.* Further work with such families has identified additional rules that emerge such as *don't think, don't question, don't ask, don't play, don't make a mistake,* etc. All of these rules stifle the health and growth of family members, promote dysfunction, and lead to family members taking on specific roles in the family in effort to cope (Black 2002).

1.1.3 Family Roles

In response to the disrupted family functioning, shifts in power, and unhealthy family rules, family members attempt to cope or "survive" the stress in the family system by adapting to a certain role. Wegscheider-Cruse's seminal roles in such families include (1) the "enabler," a caretaker who is over-responsible for others' actions; (2) the "hero," a family member who gives legitimacy to the family by finding success as others struggle to succeed; (3) the "scapegoat," the person who takes the blame for family problems and withdraws from the family as they seek attention (often negative) elsewhere; (4) the "lost child," a family member who isolates, avoids trouble, adding to a family's stress, and rarely gets any type of attention; and (5) the "mascot," a person who lessens tension in the family, covers feelings of inadequacy in the family, and provides other distraction via the use of comedy (Wegscheider-Cruse 1989). In recovery, all family roles must be given up in order for healing to take place (Wegscheider-Cruse 1989); family treatment and support groups currently aim to be supportive in this task (Shumway et al. 2017). As family roles shift back to more healthy and flexible roles in recovery, it is likely that family boundaries will also undergo change.

1.1.4 Family Boundaries

Family rules and roles ultimately help shape family boundaries, which can be thought of as demarcations of who does and does not participate in a family system. From a systemic perspective, boundaries may therefore be stated as ways in which one system is separated and can be distinguished from another, similar to how fences or property lines separate one owned piece of real estate from another (Reiter 2014). These lines of demarcation, or boundaries, in families are found in the interactions between family members, which can make them more difficult to observe and assess (Reiter 2014).

Typically, boundaries in SUD-impacted families exist on a spectrum ranging from extremes of being disengaged to "overly rigid boundaries" (Minuchin 1974). Alternatively, boundaries in healthy families are considered to be clear and flexible based on changing contexts (Minuchin 1974). Extremely rigid boundaries alter the optimal open family system, leading to a more closed system (Von Bertalanffy 1972) that is unable or unwilling to access outside help and resources. Extremely diffuse boundaries lead to enmeshment that severely restricts autonomy (Minuchin 1974) and results in chaos. For recovery to occur, it is important for extreme rigid or diffuse boundaries to shift to more clear/flexible boundaries.

1.1.5 Family Structure

Family power dynamics, rules, roles, and boundaries, among other family system dynamics, help shape a family's structure, or context/culture. This context/culture has a significant influence on the thoughts, feelings, and behaviors of individual family members. Family structures, in which an SUD is present, organize around the SUD and create a less than optimal context and environment in which all family members operate. In this way an SUD can be seen as a family disease, and recovery will require the restructuring of the family system to one that supports recovery. Such change will require challenging and reorganizing the existing family structure (Minuchin 1974) (Breakout Box 8.1).

Breakout Box 8.1. Focus on Practice

This highlight on family systems, SUD's, and family roles provide essential information for those working with families (e.g., clinicians, case managers). SUD's are complex stemming from family engagement and imitative family behaviors. As the authors identified the reality of SUD impacting family functions, personal health, and well-being, supportive research and personal recovery narratives highlight unhealthy family involvement and unhealthy well-being.

Family therapy provides a neutral role to all family members for engagement in honest and healthy dialogue regarding the impact of SUD's and unhealthy coping behaviors. Each family member can identify strengths and barriers of family functions stemming from family of origin and transferred into the family of procreation. Individuals who engage in SUD and family members impacted by SUD may experience chronic illnesses, relationship turmoil, parenting dilemmas, abuse, stress, and increased depression. Addiction is a family disease in which all members at various ages and stages of development are impacted. The family addiction disease can contribute to multiple members engaging in addictive and impulsive behavior.

The authors highlighted past research that identified the family unit influence on thoughts, feelings, and behaviors towards SUD's. Children who experience abuse and/or neglect verbally, emotionally, and physically may have negative perceptions of ability and self-worth; thus, may contribute to the likelihood of poor coping mechanisms and SUD.

Family roles, rules, and boundaries are essential to the learning of family behaviors and contributing circumstances towards SUD's. Thus, family therapy is essential towards recovery, second order change, and healthy system balance. Without positive family changes, there is an increased likelihood that family members will disengage and isolate; therefore, leading to SUD triggers and relapse.

Co-dependency and PFC factors are influenced and can contribute towards SUD's. Family members with unhealthy coping mechanisms and insufficient supportive structures may experience difficulty with healthy emotional attachment and healthy demonstrations of love, care, and support. As noted by the authors, individuals in SUD recovery need healthy support of family members. Therefore, it is essential for clinicians to provide psychoeducation, family therapy, individual processing, and community education to reduce biases and eliminate problematic contributions leading to SUD's.

– Dr. Valerie McGaha, Counseling Psychologist.

1.2 Codependency, Co-suffering, and Co-impairment

In the context of a family structure that involves unhealthy power dynamics, rules, roles, and boundaries, family members of a loved one with an SUD are considered at risk of developing a "codependency" to their loved one. Codependency involves obsession, preoccupation, and dependence (Beattie 1992; Chang 2012) regarding a loved one with an SUD. As codependent family members direct their emotional energy, time, and other efforts toward the family member with the SUD, they may neglect other things such as caring for themselves and possibly for others who may be in need of their time and attention (Daire et al. 2012). Family members with a codependency may often experience denial, overcommit themselves, and fail to keep their resolve to establish and enforce important boundaries (Dear et al. 2005). In this state, codependent family members may begin to experience their own irrational beliefs, fears of rejection, insecurities (Daire et al. 2012), the loss of a true self, and the emergence of a false self (Whitfield 2010).

These "symptoms" and suffering experienced by family members may likely be associated with the increased medical costs and claims of family members impacted by a loved one's SUD (Ray et al. 2007; Spear and Mason 1991; Weisner et al. 2010). Additionally, it is important to consider that codependency, while commonly thought of as a learned condition (Chang 2012), may involve neurological correlates associated with the stress, trauma, and pain experienced in families with a history of SUD. If so, family members may experience an impairment of how they process information and make decisions at the level of the brain, specifically the prefrontal cortex (PFC).

1.3 The Brain, Stress, and the Prefrontal Cortex

Research has shown that the brain is neurologically impacted in multiple ways by exposure to acute and chronic stress; the various structures and networks that are impacted depend on age and brain development at the time the stress occurred (Lupien et al. 2009). Additionally, the symptoms associated with such neurological impacts may be protracted, not appearing until later life stages (Lupien et al. 2009), and may also be transmitted across generations through epigenetic processes (Bale 2015; Franklin et al. 2010; Kellermann 2013; Yehuda and Lehrner 2018).

The PFC is the part of the brain responsible for the highest levels of executive functioning, including planning, decision-making (Fuster 2015), and emotional and behavioral regulation (Arnsten 2009). Exposure to stress has been shown to alter PFC structure and functioning in a negative way in prenatal, adult, and elderly/aging populations, but its impact appears to be most prominent during adolescence (Lupien et al. 2009). Glucocorticoids (stress hormones) have a neurotoxic effect on various layers of the PFC (Lupien et al. 2009) and have been associated with the retraction of dendrites (Joels et al. 2007) and reduced PFC volume (Teicher et al. 2006). Simultaneously, stress is associated with increases in volume (Lupien et al.

2009) and dendrites (Mitra et al. 2005) in the amygdala. Such alterations may be associated with the development of "bottom-up" control driven by the amygdala and other emotion-based/limbic areas in place of "top-down" control driven by PFC functioning. If so, this process is similar to dysregulation processes between the PFC and subcortical areas found with SUDs (Koob and Volkow 2016; Volkow et al. 2003; Volkow and Baler 2014). Whether considering codependency as a behavioral addiction with neurobiological correlates (Cruse and Wegscheider-Cruse 2012), or as a condition that arises as a result of stress, neuropsychology research on family members of those with an SUD is important.

1.4 Neuropsychology and PFC Functioning of SUD-Impacted Family Members

Neuropsychology research has recently been conducted regarding PFC functioning of family members of a loved one with an SUD (Shumway et al. 2019; Zielinski et al. 2019). Although these studies are preliminary and only cross-sectional in nature, they have provided some evidence suggesting altered PFC functioning of family members with an SUD loved one. Furthermore, one of these studies has shown an association between reported levels of codependency in family members and their PFC functioning in response to images of their loved one with an SUD (Zielinski et al. 2019). These preliminary studies provide a foundation for further research regarding family members, brain functioning, and codependency.

1.4.1 Altered PFC Functioning Among Family Members

Similar to how SUDs are associated with neurobiological impacts on the brain, research has hypothesized that the brains of impacted family members undergo similar changes. For example, the Impaired Response Inhibition and Salience Attribution (iRISA) syndrome regarding SUDs explains that the PFC of those with an SUD show hypoactivity in response to nonsubstance related stimuli and reinforcing cues, but hyperactivity in response to substance-related stimuli (Goldstein and Volkow 2011). This hyperactivity has shown to be most prominent in dorsolateral PFC (dlPFC) regions and is hypothesized to be associated with craving, preoccupation, and anticipation of use (Goldstein and Volkow 2011). The PFC of a concerned family member who potentially experiences codependency or "co-impairment" might be expected to show similar PFC response patterns to selected stimuli. However, the "drug-salient" cue, or trigger, for family members may be their loved one with an SUD rather than specific substance-related stimuli.

Research has recently examined this hypothesis—that family members impacted by a loved one with an SUD (experimental group) would have hyperactivation in dlPFC regions in response to images of their loved one with an SUD when compared with responses to other affective stimuli (Shumway et al. 2019). The study also hypothesized that such activation patterns would not be found in a control group (persons not experiencing SUD in their families), and that hyperactivation found in the experimental group would be more prominent in the left dlPFC (Shumway et al. 2019), given hemispheric specializations (Banich 2004) and previous SUD research (Dempsey et al. 2015).

This study utilized functional near-infrared spectroscopy (fNIR) to track cerebral blood flow (CBF—a common measure of brain activation) in the PFC as family members impacted by an SUD viewed various images, including images of their SUD loved one (see Fig. 8.1 for a representation of the PFC regions imaged by fNIR in this study). fNIR is an imaging technique growing in popularity due to low operating costs, noninvasive nature, and robust ability to manage movement artifacts (Ayaz et al. 2006). fNIR is also a unique imaging technique in that it measures both oxygenated (HbO) and deoxygenated (HbR) hemoglobin in the blood. HbO is referred to as a measure of oxygen delivery, HbR as a measure of oxygen extraction or utilization, and HbO and HbR can also be added together or subtracted from one another to create two additional CBF measures: total blood volume (HbT) and total oxygenation, respectively (Tam and Zouridakis 2014). HbR has shown to be the CBF measure most similar to the blood-oxygen-level-dependent (BOLD) signal in functional magnetic resonance imaging (fMRI) (Huppert et al. 2006).

The Shumway et al. (2019) study included 22 participants, 10 of whom were in the experimental group and 12 who comprised a control group. Experimental group participants were either a parent or spouse of a loved one with an SUD who had

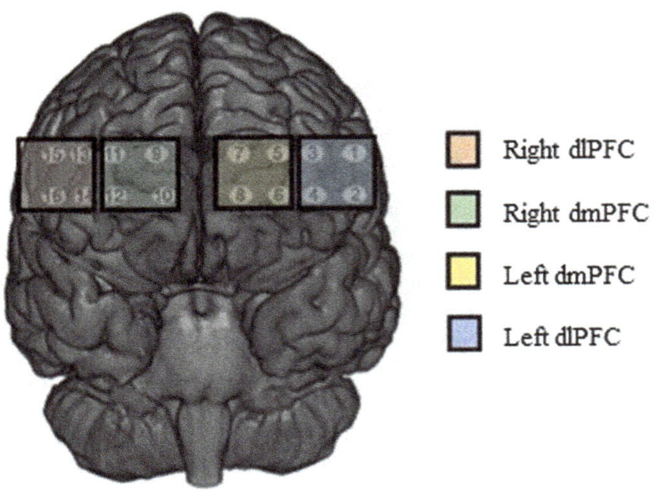

Notes: dlPFC = Dorsolateral Prefrontal Cortex
dmPFC = Dorsomedial Prefrontal Cortex
fNIR = Functional Near Infrared (Spectroscopy)

Fig. 8.1 Prefrontal cortex regions of interest measured by fNIR optodes

attended inpatient or outpatient treatment services within the previous 10 years; control group participants were similarly either a parent or spouse of a specified "target family member" with no history of SUD (see Table 8.1). Both experimental and control group participants viewed a presentation of images, including positive and negative affective images, neutral images, and images of their loved one with an SUD (or a target family member for control group participants).

Table 8.1 Descriptive statistics, experimental (n = 10) and control group (n = 12)

	Experimental group		Control group	
Variables	M (*SD*)	Min – Max	M (*SD*)	Min – Max
Age	47.90 (*16.39*)	21–70	42.25 (*12.11*)	24–62
Height (In.)	65.00 (*3.16*)	60–70	65.58 (*2.68*)	62–70
Weight (Lbs.)	*146.89 (*35.11*)	98–220	157.33 (*27.14*)	101–190
Days since loved one Tx entry	554.50 (516.95)	125–1542	*NA*	*NA*
Variables	Frequency (%)		Frequency (%)	
Gender				
Male	1 (*10*)		4 (*33.3*)	
Female	9 (*90*)		8 (*66.7*)	
Ethnicity				
Caucasian	9 (*90*)		9 (*75*)	
Hispanic	1 (*10*)		1 (*8.3*)	
Asian/Pacific Islander	NA (*NA*)		1 (*8.3*)	
Other	NA (*NA*)		1 (*8.3*)	
Education				
High school	NA (*NA*)		1 (*8.3*)	
Some college	4 (*40*)		2 (*16.7*)	
Bachelors	3 (*30*)		4 (*33.3*)	
Masters	2 (*20*)		4 (*33.3*)	
Doctoral	1 (*10*)		1 (*8.3*)	
Sexual orientation				
Heterosexual	10 (*100*)		11 (*97.7*)	
Homosexual	NA (*NA*)		1 (*8.3*)	
Relationship to loved one/target				
Family member				
Father	1 (*10*)		2 (*16.7*)	
Mother	5 (*50*)		4 (*33.3*)	
Spouse	4 (*40*)		6 (*50*)	
Religious affiliation				
Protestant	4 (*40*)		3 (*25*)	
Catholic	3 (*30*)		1 (*8.3*)	
Nondenominational	1 (*10*)		2 (*16.7*)	
Other	1 (*10*)		2 (*16.7*)	
None	1 (*10*)		4 (*33.3*)	

*n = 9 regarding weight mean for experimental group given one participant opted not to disclose

Before discussing results of the Shumway et al. (2019) study, it is important to further highlight specific regions of the PFC and some of their functions. The dlPFC regions, both left and right, are involved with important functions such as monitoring the environment, attention, working memory, and decision-making (Fuster 2015), as well as processing information related to long-term reward (Tanaka et al. 2016). In contrast, dorsomedial PFC (dmPFC) regions are involved in social cognitive processes and the development of social connections (Powers et al. 2015). The dmPFC regions have further been associated with self versus other referential processing (Vanderwal et al. 2008) as well as high level executive functioning including moral judgment, cognitive branching, and temporal processing (Greene et al. 2004).

However, left and right hemispheres of the brain are also thought to have specific specializations. For example, the left hemisphere has been associated with processing that results in "approach" behavior, while the right hemisphere with processing that results in "avoidance" behavior (Banich 2004). Thus, the right side of the brain may be more prone to err on the side of perceived risk and/or caution, and the left side to err on the side of perceived benefit. Regarding the dlPFC regions more specifically, the left dlPFC is believed to be associated with decision-making among options that have high similarity and/or explicit rules, and the right dlPFC is believed to be associated with decision-making among nonsimilar options using memory and previous experience, and/or ambiguous situations with no explicit rules (Krawczyk 2002). In a brain with healthy functioning, right and left hemispheres likely communicate via the corpus callosum when needed for complex decision-making (Banich 2004; Höller-Wallscheid et al. 2017).

Interestingly, the results from the Shumway et al. (2019) study showed significantly greater activation in both left and right dlPFC regions in response to images of the SUD loved one than in response to neutral (when utilizing HbO or oxygen delivery as a CBF measure) and positive images (when utilizing HbT or total blood volume as a CBF measure)—giving partial support to the study hypotheses (see Figs. 8.2 and 8.3). One might question if these findings mean much at all, given that an image of any family member might be more activating of PFC regions than randomly selected positive and neutral images. However, such activation patterns were not found among control group participants.

For control participants, it was the positive images that elicited a greater dlPFC activation response than that elicited by neutral images (when utilizing HbO and HbT as CBF measures). Furthermore, both positive and negative images elicited greater left dlPFC responses in control group participants than those elicited by the image of the "target family member" (when utilizing HbR as a CBF measure). In a direct comparison between experimental and control group participants, statistical analyses showed that family members in the experimental group showed lower levels of right dlPFC activation in response to images of their SUD loved one than those found among control group in response to the target family member. However, this specific difference was not hypothesized by the authors and was therefore at greater risk of being a "false positive" or statistical Type I error. A statistical adjustment called a Bonferroni correction (Bonferroni 1935) was utilized to help control

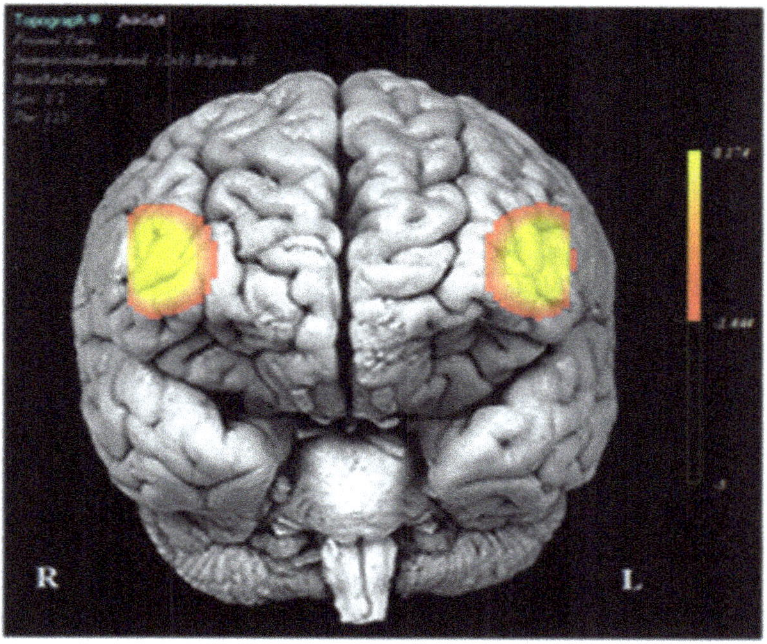

Notes: Significant differences between experimental group (N = 10) right and left dlPFC HbO activation responses to images of loved-one with a SUD and to neutral images. More specifically, this graphic shows unique activation in dlPFC regions that occurs in response to images of loved-one that does not occur in response to neutral images. Mean activation in response to neutral images was subtracted from mean activation in response to images of loved-one with SUD (including previously implemented and commonly utilized neutral subtraction). Resulting mean differences were used to map topographic image. Significant activation differences in these left and right dlPFC regions were not found among control group participants.

Fig. 8.2 Topographic representation of differences in HbO activation to images of loved one versus neutral images

the risk of claiming a significant difference when there actually is none. After this correction, the difference in right dlPFC activation was no longer considered statistically significant (Shumway et al. 2019).

The aforementioned research study provides preliminary evidence that family members impacted by the SUD of a loved one show altered neurological functioning, at least at the level of the PFC. The patterns found in this study were in some ways similar to patterns found in SUD research examining PFC responses to substance-salient cues. It can be interpreted from the results of the study that for many persons in families not impacted by SUD, images and reminders of loved ones may become somewhat common and elicit a PFC response similar to that elicited by neutral images. However, when a loved one has an SUD, PFC responses are heightened and potentially biased toward the SUD loved one.

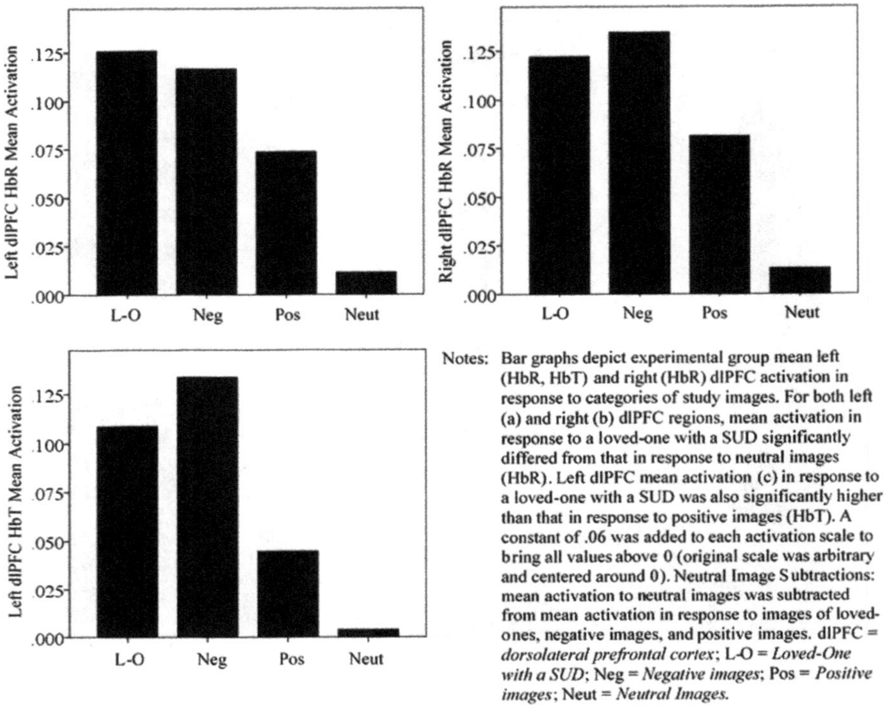

Fig. 8.3 Mean left and light dlPFC activation among experimental group in response image categories

Interestingly, it was the positive images that elicited a more heightened/biased response for control group participants. The authors suggested that this inverse finding among the control group might be preliminary—and admittedly insufficient—evidence of potential anhedonia in family members with a loved one with an SUD (experimental group). Anhedonia refers to a state in which pleasure is no longer derived from things that were once pleasurable (Loas 1996). Anhedonia is often a condition associated with having an SUD as well as other mental health conditions such as depression, both conditions for which family members of a loved one with an SUD have heightened risk (Ray et al. 2007). However, what is not fully clear is whether or not the alterations of PFC functioning found in this study reflect more than some type of "codependency" similar to an SUD, such as potential results from the stress and fear often found in situations associated with SUD. Such an effect on the brain may be similar to that found in those with a history of trauma (Carrion and Wong 2012). Importantly, additional research has found association between reported levels of codependency and PFC functioning.

1.4.2 Codependency and PFC Functioning

Another study using the same methods as the previously mentioned study (Shumway et al. 2019) examined the relationship between codependency and family member PFC activation patterns in response to images of a loved one with an SUD (Zielinski et al. 2019). However, this study involved a larger sample (n = 26) that included siblings (n = 8), a significant other (n = 1), and other close family members (e.g., grandparents, n = 7) in addition to parents and spouses (n = 10). Again, activation for this experimental group was compared against that of a control group comprised of parents and spouses of a "target family member" and confirmed no diagnosed SUD for themselves or within their family for three generations (see Table 8.2).

All participants in this study responded to the Spann-Fischer Codependency Scale (Fischer and Spann 1991). Those in the experimental group reported clinically moderate and significantly higher levels of codependency compared to relatively low clinical levels reported by the control group. For the experimental group, codependency significantly correlated with decreased activation in the left dmPFC in response to images of their SUD-loved one (see Figs. 8.4 and 8.5). This negative relationship between codependency and left dmPFC activation in the experimental group was significantly larger than this same relationship in the control group and was also significantly larger than the relationships between codependency and left dmPFC activation responses to negative and neutral images.

The left dmPFC, along with other regions of the PFC, has been associated with some of the highest levels of executive functioning, such as goal setting and processing information regarding important relationships (Eickhoff et al. 2014). This region of the PFC therefore, plays an important role in the development of social connections (Powers et al. 2015) and is involved when information from past social interactions is processed to form current responses to social situations (Spreng et al. 2009). Knowing this, Zielinski et al. (2019) inferred that this region of the PFC is important for family members when making decisions in emotional situations regarding their loved one suffering from an SUD. Inversely, reduced activation in this region may be associated with diminished ability to make proactive decisions of which the consequences and potential outcomes have been carefully considered.

In another neuropsychology study, Pochon et al. (2002) suggested that decreased activation in the left dmPFC maybe not only involved with reduced cognitive demand and executive function, but also with attempts to avoid emotional information associated with anxiety and/or fear of failure. Therefore, reduced activation in this region associating with codependency may reflect processing that excludes information about how a certain action may lead to an undesired or unintended outcome, or that is associated with feelings of failure, fear, or hopelessness. If so, reduced activation in the left dmPFC associated with codependency may be in part an explanation of "enabling" behaviors that ultimately maintain SUD patterns (Zielinski et al. 2019).

Table 8.2 Descriptive statistics, experimental (n = 26) and control group (n = 12)

	Experimental group		Control group	
Variables	M (*SD*)	Min – Max	M (*SD*)	Min – Max
[a]Age	32.58 (*16.27*)	18–70	42.25 (*12.11*)	24–62
Days since loved one treatment entry	384.27 (369.55)	7–1542	*NA*	*NA*
Variables	Frequency (%)		Frequency (%)	
Gender				
Male	4 (*15.4*)		4 (*33.3*)	
Female	22 (*84.6*)		8 (*66.7*)	
Ethnicity				
Caucasian	23 (*88.5*)		9 (*75*)	
African American	1 (*3.8*)		1 (*8.3*)	
Hispanic	2 (*7.7*)		1 (*8.3*)	
Asian/Pacific Islander	*NA*		1 (*8.3*)	
Other	*NA*		1 (*8.3*)	
Education				
High school	1 (*3.8*)		1 (*8.3*)	
Some college	14 (*53.8*)		2 (*16.7*)	
Bachelors	4 (*15.4*)		4 (*33.3*)	
Masters	6 (*23.1*)		4 (*33.3*)	
Doctoral	1 (*3.8*)		1 (*8.3*)	
Sexual orientation				
Heterosexual	25 (*96.2*)		11 (*91.7*)	
Homosexual	1 (*3.8*)		1 (*8.3*)	
Relationship to loved one/target				
Family member				
Father	1 (*3.8*)		2 (*16.7*)	
Mother	5 (*19.2*)		4 (*33.3*)	
Spouse	4 (*15.4*)		6 (*50*)	
Significant other	1 (*3.8*)		*NA*	
Sibling	8 (*30.8*)		*NA*	
Other	7 (*26.9*)		*NA*	
Religious affiliation				
Protestant	7 (*26.9*)		3 (*25*)	
Catholic	4 (*15.4*)		1 (*8.3*)	
Nondenominational	8 (*30.8*)		2 (*16.7*)	
Other	3 (*11.5*)		2 (*16.7*)	
None	4 (*15.4*)		4 (*33.3*)	

[a]Was not significantly different at $p < 0.05$ when assuming equal variances (however, p = 0.05 when unequal variances are assumed)

The Zielinski et al. (2019) study on codependency also highlighted that research has shown an association between increased dmPFC activation and empathic inferences as well as altruistic and prosocial behavior (Waytz et al. 2012). Therefore, reduced dmPFC activation found in this study could suggest that family members

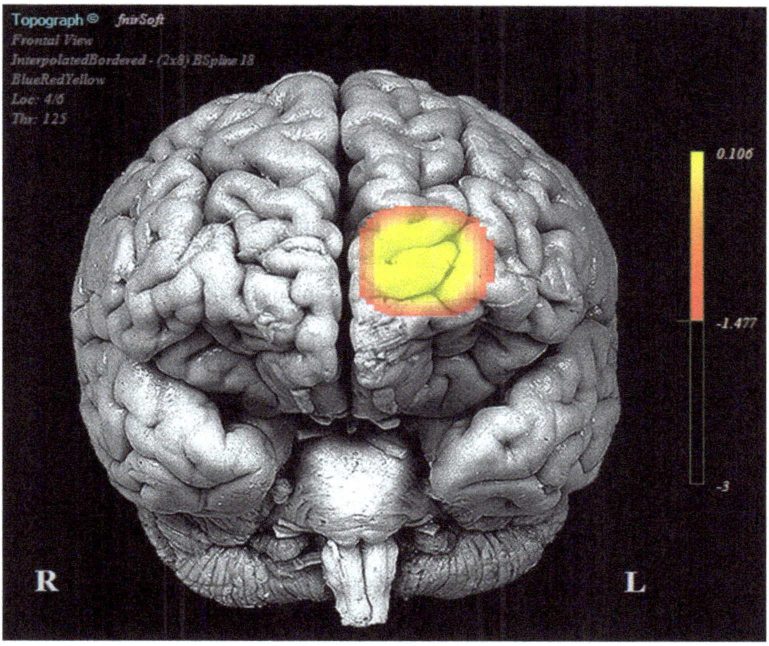

Notes: Significant left dmPFC activation unique to low levels of codependency when viewing images of a loved-one with a SUD in the experimental group. Average activation for the left dmPFC of experimental group participants in a high codependency group ($N = 8$) was subtracted from average left dmPFC activation of participants in a low codependency group ($N = 9$), while viewing images of a loved-one with a SUD. For visualization purposes, a middle level codependency group ($N = 9$) was not included in the topographic image.

dmPFC = dorsomedial prefrontal cortex

Fig. 8.4 Topographic representation of activation differences to images of SUD loved one for low and high codependency

with higher levels of codependency may have somewhat altered perceptions about what is truly best for their loved one and their potential recovery, and their efforts to help could have unintended, counteractive effects (Zielinski et al. 2019). However, it was noted in this study that research has shown that chronic illness in general can have a strong and negative impact on caring and concerned family members (Rolland 1993), and the results found may not be specific to SUD-related impacts but rather to chronic illnesses in general (Zielinski et al. 2019).

Family members impacted by the SUD of a loved one are in need of personal recovery. Their own recovery can have positive impacts on not only their own health but also that of the entire family system (Steinglass 1985). The results of this study also suggest that the support and resources family members may need extend deeper than brief inclusion in treatment that invites family members to change "enabling"

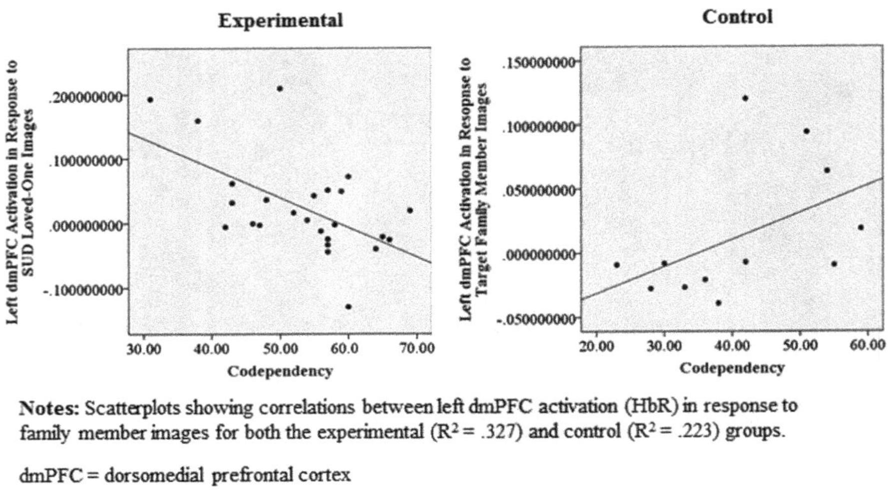

Fig. 8.5 Scatterplots of lDMPFC activation in response to family member cues and SFCS totals

behaviors. However, family members may often not be aware of or have available resources that promote their recovery. It is important for clinicians and other professionals to aid family members in finding social support and other resources that promote healthy coping skills and individual recovery (Zielinski et al. 2019). Such resources could play a vital role in their recovery as they may aid the family members in several ways to make important decisions that impact both the recovery of their SUD-love and their own recovery. Supportive relationships are a vital element of recovery for those with an SUD (Laudet et al. 2006), and they can often find experience, strength, hope (Bradley 2011), support, reassurance, and direction from others as they seek recovery. Family members may similarly find reassurance, hope, comfort, and direction as they engage with others.

Alanon is one example of a support group that research has shown offers family members support in the recovery process. This support groups include various mechanisms that support family members in managing the "uncertainty" and lack of power in the recovery process (Kuuluvainen and Isotalus 2015). Family members finding recovery often have to shift their focus toward themselves and their own well-being (Shumway et al. 2017), and in the process face uncertainty regarding many things, including whether or not their loved one with the SUD will abstain and find successful recovery. This example of social support is important regarding the relationship found between codependency and reduced left dmPFC activation as this region of the PFC has also been shown to play an important role in the cognitive processing of uncertainty (Bzdok et al. 2013). A supportive network of relationships can also share perspective regarding decisions that family members make or plan to make.

1.5 Implications

1.5.1 Implications for Understanding Family Resilience

Resilience is difficult to define, and while there is not a consensus definition, research has identified key themes associated with resilience, including rising above to overcome adversity, adaptation and adjustment, 'ordinary magic', good mental health, and the ability to bounce back (Aburn et al. 2016). While many of these themes are somewhat self-evident, "ordinary magic" refers to the idea that resiliency is grounded in everyday, ordinary things in the lived experience, and like magic, it is difficult to measure (Masten 2001). While resilience for a significant period of time was thought of as an individual characteristic or capacity, a recognition of families as resilient with a similar ability to grow, adapt, and become stronger through adversity has emerged and developed (Walsh 2003). Understanding SUDs as a "family disease" (Roth 2010) or condition in which family members also experience "co-impairment" and are in need of individual recovery during a family recovery process is not a demeaning or pejorative perspective. On the contrary, such a systemic perspective views the family as a strong, adaptive, and resourceful system that helps weather a storm of illness and has a capacity to be the most important support structure in recovery.

The shifts in power dynamics, rules, roles, and boundaries that alter family structure during the course of an SUD also demonstrate adaptability in the family. While these shifts are not sustainable and lead to a decline of health over the long term, early scholars studying families experiencing alcoholism recognized them as attempts at survival (Brown and Lewis 1995). For example, family roles that develop under such conditions have been termed *Survival Roles* (Black 1992). Black (1992) also describes family rules that ultimately lead to more of a closed system as attempts to survive the current stresses often found in families experiencing an SUD. Ultimately, while these shifts lead to pain and health limitations, they help the family survive and manage acute situations of stress until further resources and direction might be found and implemented. It is important to consider that resiliency is a process and not just a momentary capacity (Walsh 2003), and that changes in family structure during SUD development can be considered part of a resiliency process that involves the need for additional change during recovery.

1.5.2 Implications for Practice and/or Policy

Research on SUDs has largely been comprised of work on with the index SUD case, with limited attention to biological, psychological, and social factors involving impacted family members (Orford et al. 2010). Discussion regarding the family unit and SUDs is now becoming common and often includes the concept of codependency and behaviors that enable problematic substance use to continue (Whitfield 2010). Some research has examined codependency and suggested that it may be associated with personality (Hoenigmann-Lion and Whitehead 2007). Nevertheless, complexity remains regarding family systems that are impacted by SUDs and the resulting behaviors and patterns of interaction that emerge. Research examining neurological patterns of altered function has begun to explore such complexity (Shumway et al. 2019; Zielinski et al. 2019). These previously discussed studies illustrate the importance of providing family members with additional attention, support, resources, and even treatments that might aid them in finding personal recovery. These neurological impacts may alter thinking, perception, and behaviors that ultimately will negatively influence individual health as well as the family as a system of support. Family members should be involved and not overlooked during recovery processes.

Previous research on aspects of the family system and family recovery process has suggested that individual recovery for family members is the most important priority during early recovery, while family and relationship recovery may better occur in more moderate or long-term recovery stages (Brown and Lewis 1995). Multifamily groups, however, are now fairly commonplace in early stages of SUD treatment, and research on these groups suggests that aspects of family functioning and relationship recovery may be important throughout the recovery process (Shumway et al. 2017). However, individual recovery is important in parallel to family and relationship recovery, and caution should be taken as to how this might most effectively be accomplished (Bradshaw et al. 2016; Shumway et al. 2019). Shumway et al. (2017) found important benefits of family involvement in the early recovery process as a result of a multifamily group intervention; however, some of these benefits were reduced or even lost over time. Involving family and working on relationships in early recovery stages can be effective, but more efforts are needed to provide family members with continued attention and support beyond the initial involvement currently found in many treatment settings (Shumway et al. 2017).

1.6 Conclusion and Future Directions

1.6.1 Concluding Remarks

Taking the perspective of families as a systemic unit opens greater possibilities for understanding the development of and recovery from an SUD. As the understanding of the reciprocal impact of individual family members on the family atmosphere and that atmosphere on the individual continues to develop, so might new and effective treatments that support and sustain recovery. Family members experience much stress, and the family undergoes other challenging circumstances, which increases risk of poor physical and mental health outcomes. The research discussed in this chapter suggests that family members may experience neurological changes that affect PFC functioning. While self-help support structures and networks are available in support of families impacted by an SUD, many other resources can be financially or geographically unavailable, or remain nonexistent and are yet to be developed. Continued focus on the family in the recovery process can promote such developments.

1.6.2 Considerations Moving Forward

In terms of future research, both the Shumway et al. (2019) and Zielinski et al. (2019) studies acknowledge important limitations to be considered by future research. For example, the samples of these studies were limited both in size and by a lack of ethnic diversity, and research that examines similar phenomenon in larger and more ethnically diverse samples is important. Additionally, the control group for these studies was not ideally matched as could be hoped for, another consideration for future research. Additionally, fMRI imaging techniques can measure activation in subcortical brain regions and would be extremely beneficial to further corroborate the findings of these studies, as would research that utilizes carefully designed longitudinal methods. Furthermore, examining family member's or caregiver's brain activation responses to images of family members with other types of chronic illness, as well as images of another family member who does not have an SUD or chronic illness, would also help further substantiate this preliminary research.

Clinical and organizational changes may continue to occur as well. Treatment centers may find new and enhanced ways to involve family members, and for longer durations. Insurance companies may evaluate policies and procedures in hopes to provide greater availability of resources to families, which over time may also be more cost-effective. Overall, there is reason to be optimistic for the future as it relates to families facing the challenge and opportunity of finding recovery from SUD. The resilience of these families and providers who make efforts to serve and support them is inspiring and encouraging.

Glossary of Terms

Family (system) an emotional unit, an entity in its own right with principles of operation that regulate the functioning of the entity's parts (Kerr et al. 1988)

Substance Use Disorder a problematic pattern of use of an intoxicating substance leading to clinically significant impairment or distress with 10 or 11 diagnostic criteria (depending on the substance) occurring within a 12-month period (DSM V)

Codependency any combination of dependence, obsession, and preoccupation toward another person (Zielinski et al. 2019)—often a person with an SUD or mental health disorder; one who has let another person's behavior affect him or her, and who is obsessed with controlling that person's behavior (Beattie 1992)

Recovery a regenerative and transformative growth process from addictive behavior that nurtures a sustainable lifestyle of hope and resiliency. A recovery lifestyle is evidenced by positive identity and worth, healthy coping skills, meaningful relationships, purpose-driven achievements and accomplishments, and results in expanded choice and opportunity.

Prefrontal Cortex the cortex of the anterior pole of the mammalian brain; the part of the cerebral cortex that receives projections from the mediodorsal nucleus of the thalamus, with the basic function of representation and execution of new forms of organized goal-directed action (Fuster 2015, p. 1)

System an integrated whole whose essential properties arise from the relationships between its parts and "systems thinking" [is] the understanding of a phenomenon within the context of a larger whole (Capra and Luisi 2014, p. 64)

Treatment any intervention by recognized programs or individuals whose primary goal is to treat individuals with substance use problems (Klingemann et al. 2001)

Questions for Thought and Discussion

1. What are feasible ways that the existing addiction and mental health system of care may be altered to provide greater continued support for family members?
2. How can research examine differences between codependency or "co-impairment" and the common effects that occur as a result of traumatic stress?
3. Does an SUD in the family lead to the results found in the studies highlighted in this chapter, or do intergenerational patterns and/or preexisting conditions in families potentially precede SUD development? What longitudinal research methods might answer this question?
4. What are some of the most common obstacles that inhibit family members from having personal treatment and resources that aid them in their own recovery?
5. Is it possible for the individualized health care system to shift to a more balanced paradigm that involves a greater collectivistic focus? What might precede or encourage such a shift?

References

Aburn, G., Gott, M., & Hoare, K. (2016). What is resilience? An integrative review of the empirical literature. *Journal of Advanced Nursing, 72*(5), 980–1000.

Alcoholics Anonymous (4th ed.). (2001). Alcoholics Anonymous World Services, Inc.

Arnsten, A. F. (2009). Stress signalling pathways that impair prefrontal cortex structure and function. *Nature Reviews Neuroscience, 10*(6), 410.

Ayaz, H., Izzetoglu, M., Platek, S. M., Bunce, S., Izzetoglu, K., Pourrezaei, K., & Onaral, B. (2006). Registering fNIR data to brain surface image using MRI templates. In *Engineering in medicine and biology society, 2006. EMBS'06. 28th annual international conference of the IEEE*, pp. 2671–2674.

Bale, T. L. (2015). Epigenetic and transgenerational reprogramming of brain development. *Nature Reviews Neuroscience, 16*(6), 332.

Banich, M. T. (2004). *Cognitive neuroscience and neuropsychology* (2nd ed.). Boston: Houghton Mifflin.

Beattie, M. (1992). *Codependent no more: How to stop controlling others and start caring for yourself.* Center City: Hazelden Publishing.

Black, C. (1992). *Effects of family alcoholism. Alcoholism and the Family*, 272–281.

Black, C. (2002). *It will never happen to me: Growing up with addiction as youngsters, adolescents, adults*. Center City: Hazelden Publishing.

Bonferroni, C. E. (1935). *Il calcolo delle assicurazioni su gruppi di teste. Studi in Onore Del Professore Salvatore Ortu Carboni*, 13–60.

Bradley, C. A. (2011). Women in AA: "Sharing experience, strength and hope" the relational nature of spirituality. *Journal of Religion & Spirituality in Social Work: Social Thought, 30*(2), 89–112.

Bradshaw, S. D., Shumway, S. T., Wang, E. W., Harris, K. S., Smith, D. B., & Austin-Robillard, H. (2016). Family functioning and readiness in family recovery from addiction. *Journal of Groups in Addiction & Recovery, 11*(1), 21–41.

Broderick, C. B. (1993). *Understanding family process: Basics of family systems theory*. London: Sage.

Broderick, C., & Smith, J. (n.d.). *The general systems approach to the family.*

Brown, S., & Lewis, V. (1995). The alcoholic family: A developmental model of recovery. In *Treating alcoholism*. San Francisco: Josey Bass.

Bzdok, D., Langner, R., Schilbach, L., Engemann, D. A., Laird, A. R., Fox, P. T., & Eickhoff, S. (2013). Segregation of the human medial prefrontal cortex in social cognition. *Frontiers in Human Neuroscience, 7*, 232.

Capra, F., & Luisi, P. L. (2014). *The systems view of life: A unifying vision*. Cambridge: Cambridge University Press.

Carrion, V. G., & Wong, S. S. (2012). Can traumatic stress alter the brain? Understanding the implications of early trauma on brain development and learning. *Journal of Adolescent Health, 51*(2), S23–S28.

Chang, S.-H. (2012). A cultural perspective on codependency and its treatment. *Asia Pacific Journal of Counselling and Psychotherapy, 3*(1), 50–60.

Cruse, J., & Wegscheider-Cruse, S. (2012). *Understanding codependency, updated and expanded: The science behind it and how to break the cycle*. Health Communications, Inc.

Daire, A. P., Jacobson, L., & Carlson, R. G. (2012). Emotional stocks and bonds: A metaphorical model for conceptualizing and treating codependency and other forms of emotional overinvesting. *American Journal of Psychotherapy, 66*(3), 259–278.

Dear, G. E., Roberts, C. M., & Lange, L. (2005). *Defining codependency: A thematic analysis of published definitions*.

Dempsey, J. P., Harris, K. S., Shumway, S. T., Kimball, T. G., Herrera, J. C., Dsauza, C. M., & Bradshaw, S. D. (2015). Functional near infrared spectroscopy as a potential biological assessment of addiction recovery: Preliminary findings. *The American Journal of Drug and Alcohol Abuse, 41*(2), 119–126.

Eickhoff, S. B., Laird, A. R., Fox, P. T., Bzdok, D., & Hensel, L. (2014). Functional segregation of the human dorsomedial prefrontal cortex. *Cerebral Cortex, 26*(1), 304–321.

England Kennedy, E. S., & Horton, S. (2011). "Everything that I thought that they would be, they weren't:" Family systems as support and impediment to recovery. *Social Science & Medicine, 73*(8), 1222–1229.

Fischer, J. L., & Spann, L. (1991). Measuring codependency. *Alcoholism Treatment Quarterly, 8*(1), 87–100.

Franklin, T. B., Russig, H., Weiss, I. C., Gräff, J., Linder, N., Michalon, A., Vizi, S., & Mansuy, I. M. (2010). Epigenetic transmission of the impact of early stress across generations. *Biological Psychiatry, 68*(5), 408–415.

Fuster, J. (2015). *The prefrontal cortex*. Amsterdam: Academic.

Goldstein, R. Z., & Volkow, N. D. (2011). Dysfunction of the prefrontal cortex in addiction: Neuroimaging findings and clinical implications. *Nature Reviews Neuroscience, 12*(11), 652.

Greene, J. D., Nystrom, L. E., Engell, A. D., Darley, J. M., & Cohen, J. D. (2004). The neural bases of cognitive conflict and control in moral judgment. *Neuron, 44*(2), 389–400.

Hoenigmann-Lion, N. M., & Whitehead, G. I. (2007). The relationship between codependency and borderline and dependent personality traits. *Alcoholism Treatment Quarterly, 24*(4), 55–77.

Höller-Wallscheid, M. S., Thier, P., Pomper, J. K., & Lindner, A. (2017). Bilateral recruitment of prefrontal cortex in working memory is associated with task demand but not with age. *Proceedings of the National Academy of Sciences, 114*(5), E830–E839. https://doi.org/10.1073/pnas.1601983114.

How Al-Anon Works for Families and Friends of Alcoholics. (1995). Al-Anon Family Groups.

Huppert, T. J., Hoge, R. D., Diamond, S. G., Franceschini, M. A., & Boas, D. A. (2006). A temporal comparison of BOLD, ASL, and NIRS hemodynamic responses to motor stimuli in adult humans. *NeuroImage, 29*(2), 368–382. https://doi.org/10.1016/j.neuroimage.2005.08.065.

Joels, M., Karst, H., Krugers, H. J., & Lucassen, P. J. (2007). Chronic stress: Implications for neuronal morphology, function and neurogenesis. *Frontiers in Neuroendocrinology, 28*(2–3), 72–96.

Kellermann, N. P. (2013). Epigenetic transmission of holocaust trauma: Can nightmares be inherited. *The Israel Journal of Psychiatry and Related Sciences, 50*(1), 33–39.

Kerr, M. E., Bowen, M., & Kerr, M. E. (1988). *Family evaluation*. New York: WW Norton & Company.

Klingemann, H., Sobell, L. C., Barker, J., Blomqvist, J., Cloud, W., Ellinstad, T., et al. (2001). *Promoting self-change from problem substance use: Practical implications for policy, prevention and treatment*. Springer Science & Business Media.

Koob, G. F., & Volkow, N. D. (2016). Neurobiology of addiction: A neurocircuitry analysis. *The Lancet Psychiatry, 3*(8), 760–773.

Krawczyk, D. C. (2002). Contributions of the prefrontal cortex to the neural basis of human decision making. *Neuroscience & Biobehavioral Reviews, 26*(6), 631–664.

Krestan, J. (2000). *Addiction, power, and powerlessness. Bridges to recovery: Addiction, family therapy & multicultural treatment*, 15–44.

Kuuluvainen, V., & Isotalus, P. (2015). Words and beyond: Members' experiences of the supportive communication and helping mechanisms of Al-anon groups. *Journal of Groups in Addiction & Recovery, 10*(3), 204–223.

Laudet, A. B., Morgen, K., & White, W. L. (2006). The role of social supports, spirituality, religiousness, life meaning and affiliation with 12-step fellowships in quality of life satisfaction among individuals in recovery from alcohol and drug problems. *Alcoholism Treatment Quarterly, 24*(1–2), 33–73.

Loas, G. (1996). Vulnerability to depression: A model centered on anhedonia. *Journal of Affective Disorders, 41*(1), 39–53.

Lupien, S. J., McEwen, B. S., Gunnar, M. R., & Heim, C. (2009). Effects of stress throughout the lifespan on the brain, behaviour and cognition. *Nature Reviews Neuroscience, 10*(6), 434.

Masten, A. S. (2001). Ordinary magic: Resilience processes in development. *American Psychologist, 56*(3), 227.

McEwen, B. S. (2012). Brain on stress: How the social environment gets under the skin. *Proceedings of the National Academy of Sciences, 109*(Supplement 2), 17180–17185.

Minuchin, S. (1974). *Families & family therapy (1974-21519-000)*. Cambridge: Harvard University Press.

Mitra, R., Jadhav, S., McEwen, B. S., Vyas, A., & Chattarji, S. (2005). Stress duration modulates the spatiotemporal patterns of spine formation in the basolateral amygdala. *Proceedings of the National Academy of Sciences, 102*(26), 9371–9376.

Moos, R. H., & Moos, B. S. (1984). The process of recovery from alcoholism: III. Comparing functioning in families of alcoholics and matched control families. *Journal of Studies on Alcohol, 45*(2), 111–118.

Orford, J., Templeton, L., Velleman, R., & Copello, A. (2010). Methods of assessment for affected family members. *Drugs: Education, Prevention and Policy, 17*(sup1), 75–85.

Orford, J., Velleman, R., Natera, G., Templeton, L., & Copello, A. (2013). Addiction in the family is a major but neglected contributor to the global burden of adult ill-health. *Social Science & Medicine, 78*, 70–77.

Pochon, J. B., Levy, R., Fossati, P., Lehericy, S., Poline, J. B., Pillon, B., Le Bihan, D., & Dubois, B. (2002). The neural system that bridges reward and cognition in humans: An fMRI study. *Proceedings of the National Academy of Sciences, 99*(8), 5669–5674.

Powers, K. E., Chavez, R. S., & Heatherton, T. F. (2015). Individual differences in response of dorsomedial prefrontal cortex predict daily social behavior. *Social Cognitive and Affective Neuroscience, 11*(1), 121–126.

Ray, G. T., Mertens, J. R., & Weisner, C. (2007). The excess medical cost and health problems of family members of persons diagnosed with alcohol or drug problems. *Medical Care, 45*(2), 116–122.

Reiter, M. D. (2014). *Substance abuse and the family*. New York: Routledge.

Rolland, J. S. (1993). Mastering family challenges in serious illness and disability. *Normal Family Processes, 2*, 444–473.

Roth, J. D. (2010). *Addiction as a family disease*. Philadelphia: Taylor & Francis.

Schäfer, G. (2011). Family functioning in families with alcohol and other drug addiction. *Social Policy Journal of New Zealand, 37*(2), 135–151.

Schwartz, R. C., & Nichols, M. P. (2004). *Family therapy: Concepts and methods*. Boston: Pearson Allyn and Bacon.

Shumway, S. T., Schonian, S., Bradshaw, S., & Hayes, N. D. (2017). A revised multifamily group curriculum: The need for family member recovery from addiction. *Journal of Groups in Addiction & Recovery, 12*(4), 260–283.

Shumway, S. T., Bradshaw, S. D., Hayes, N., Schonian, S., & Kimball, T. G. (2019). Prefrontal cortex functioning of family members of those with a substance use disorder. *Alcoholism Treatment Quarterly, 37*(1), 75–98.

Spear, S. F., & Mason, M. (1991). Impact of chemical dependency on family health status. *International Journal of the Addictions, 26*(2), 179–187.

Spreng, R. N., Mar, R. A., & Kim, A. S. (2009). The common neural basis of autobiographical memory, prospection, navigation, theory of mind, and the default mode: A quantitative meta-analysis. *Journal of Cognitive Neuroscience, 21*(3), 489–510.

Steinglass, P. (1985). Family systems approaches to alcoholism. *Journal of Substance Abuse Treatment, 2*(3), 161–167.

Tam, N. D., & Zouridakis, G. (2014). Temporal decoupling of oxy-and deoxy-hemoglobin hemodynamic responses detected by functional near-infrared spectroscopy (fNIRS). *Journal of Biomedical Engineering and Medical Imaging, 1*(2), 18–28.

Tanaka, S. C., Doya, K., Okada, G., Ueda, K., Okamoto, Y., & Yamawaki, S. (2016). Prediction of immediate and future rewards differentially recruits cortico-basal ganglia loops. In *Behavioral economics of preferences, choices, and happiness* (pp. 593–616). Tokyo: Springer.

Teicher, M. H., Tomoda, A., & Andersen, S. L. (2006). Neurobiological consequences of early stress and childhood maltreatment: Are results from human and animal studies comparable? *Annals of the New York Academy of Sciences, 1071*(1), 313–323.

Vanderwal, T., Hunyadi, E., Grupe, D. W., Connors, C. M., & Schultz, R. T. (2008). Self, mother and abstract other: An fMRI study of reflective social processing. *NeuroImage, 41*(4), 1437–1446. https://doi.org/10.1016/j.neuroimage.2008.03.058.

Volkow, N. D., & Baler, R. D. (2014). Addiction science: Uncovering neurobiological complexity. *Neuropharmacology, 76*, 235–249.

Volkow, N. D., Fowler, J. S., & Wang, G.-J. (2003). The addicted human brain: Insights from imaging studies. *The Journal of Clinical Investigation, 111*(10), 1444–1451.

Von Bertalanffy, L. (1972). The history and status of general systems theory. *Academy of Management Journal, 15*(4), 407–426.

Walsh, F. (2003). Family resilience: A framework for clinical practice. *Family Process, 42*(1), 1–18.

Waytz, A., Zaki, J., & Mitchell, J. P. (2012). Response of dorsomedial prefrontal cortex predicts altruistic behavior. *Journal of Neuroscience, 32*(22), 7646–7650.

Wegscheider-Cruse, S. (1989). *Another chance: Hope and health for the alcoholic family*. Palo Alto: Science & Behavior Books.

Weisner, C., Parthasarathy, S., Moore, C., & Mertens, J. R. (2010). Individuals receiving addiction treatment: Are medical costs of their family members reduced? *Addiction, 105*(7), 1226–1234.

Whitfield, C. (2010). *Co-dependence healing the human condition: The new paradigm for helping professionals and people in recovery*. Simon and Schuster.

Yehuda, R., & Lehrner, A. (2018). Intergenerational transmission of trauma effects: Putative role of epigenetic mechanisms. *World Psychiatry, 17*(3), 243–257.

Zielinski, M., Bradshaw, S., Mullet, N., Hawkins, L., Shumway, S., & Story Chavez, M. (2019). Codependency and prefrontal cortex functioning: Preliminary examination of substance use disorder impacted family members. *The American Journal on Addictions, 28*, 367–375.

Index

J. M. Croff, J. Beaman (eds.), *Family Resilience and Recovery from Opioids and Other Addictions*, Emerging Issues in Family and Individual Resilience,
https://doi.org/10.1007/978-3-030-56958-7

www.ingramcontent.com/pod-product-compliance
Lightning Source LLC
Chambersburg PA
CBHW071143040926
50963CB00003B/156
9783030569570